Salma NSIRI
Khédija SOUMER

Evolutionary profile of tricuspid lesions after left heart surgery

Salma NSIRI
Khédija SOUMER

Evolutionary profile of tricuspid lesions after left heart surgery

Long-term results and factors associated with aggravation

ScienciaScripts

Cover image: www.ingimage.com

This book is a translation from the original published under ISBN 978-620-6-71921-2.

Publisher:
Sciencia Scripts
is a trademark of
Dodo Books Indian Ocean Ltd. and OmniScriptum S.R.L publishing group

120 High Road, East Finchley, London, N2 9ED, United Kingdom
Str. Armeneasca 28/1, office 1, Chisinau MD-2012, Republic of Moldova, Europe
Managing Directors: Ieva Konstantinova, Victoria Ursu
info@omniscriptum.com

Printed at: see last page
ISBN: 978-620-8-59442-8

Contents

To my dearest parents,

My mother Leila and my father Abdelfatteh,

All the words in the world cannot express the immense love I feel for you

love I feel for you, nor the deep gratitude I feel for all your

for all your efforts and sacrifices.

You have always believed in me and your encouragement has never stopped

to push me forward

I want you to be proud of me, and I want you to know that I've lived up to the hopes

you had for me.

hopes you had for me

As a token of my affection and gratitude, allow me to thank you through this work.

through this work to thank you.

May God preserve you good health and long life

I love you all.

To my brother A mir and my sisters A mira, Jalil a and Jihen,

You know that my love for you knows no bounds.

You've never stopped encouraging me and supporting me every step of the way.

May we remain united in tenderness and faithful to the education

we have received

I pray that God will bring you happiness and help you to realise your

dreams.

I dedicate this work to you as a token of my love.

To my dear Nour and Mehdi,

My little niece and nephew, your presence lights up our lives

Every moment spent with you is an immense joy and I'm looking forward

to be an auntie

This work is proof of my eternal love for you

May happiness be with you all life

To my dear aunt Halima and my dear cousin Mariem,

Words cannot express all my gratitude and love.

my love

Your generosity and support have really helped me to move forward

forward

This work shows my love and gratitude

To my confidant Hazem,

I will always be grateful for all the encouragement, respect and love

respect and love you have given me

Thank you for your unconditional support, your optimism and your infinite patience.

patience.

I dedicate this work to you as a token of my love and complicity.

To my very dear friends

Those who have supported me without limits, those who have helped me and who

have
in good times and bad
Thank you for being my source of motivation and happiness.
My special thanks go to all those who contributed to this work.
this work.
You will find in it the expression of my most sincere gratitude and affection.

Acknowledgements

To our Master and President of the jury
Professor Amine JEMEL
Head of Cardiovascular Surgery
CHU Abderrahmen Mami

We would like to thank you for the honour you have done us in agreeing agreeing to chair our thesis jury

We will always have the utmost respect for your kindness, your kindness and your human and professional qualities. and professional qualities.

Your competence, your dynamism, your clear and precise teaching and precise teaching, and your rigorous approach to your work have always admiration and high esteem.

Please find in this work, dear master, the testimony of our sincere gratitude and the assurance of our highest consideration.

To our Master and Judge
Professor Sonia OUERGHI
Department of Anaesthesia and Intensive Care
CHU Abderrahmen Mami

We are very touched by the honour you have done us in agreeing agreeing to judge this thesis

Your skill, professional rigour and distinguished human qualities have always human qualities have always commanded our deepest admiration. admiration

Please find in this work the expression of our great admiration admiration and deep gratitude

To our Master and Judge
Professor Henda NEJI
Medical Imaging Department
CHU Abderrahmen Mami

You are doing us a great honour by agreeing to sit on our esteemed jury

We admire your competence, your seriousness and your human and professional qualities. and professional qualities

We would like to take this opportunity to express to you, dear master our deepest gratitude and respect for your work.

To our Master and Judge
Professor Mouna BOUSNIN A
Department of Cardiovascular Surgery
CHU Abderrahmen Mami

Thank you very much for agreeing to judge our thesis, and we are deeply grateful to you

Your rigour, your competence, your human and professional qualities

and professional qualities can only arouse esteem and respect
Your generosity and invaluable advice will always be with us.
Please find in this work the expression of our great admiration
admiration and our deepest gratitude

To our Master and Judge
Professor Emna BEN NOUR
Cardiology Department
CHU Abderrahmen Mami

We are very honoured that you have agreed to sit on our jury.
members of our jury
Your human and professional qualities command our deep respect and
respect and admiration
We would like to thank you for your kindness, your attentiveness and your
advice that will never be forgotten
May this work be a token of our sincerest and deepest gratitude
and deepest gratitude

To our Master and Thesis Reporter
Professor Mokhles LAJMI
Department of Cardiovascular Surgery
Tunis Military Hospital

It is a great honour for you to agree to report on this work.
Your kindness, your generosity and your knowledge have always aroused
our great admiration
Your availability, your advice and your invaluable comments were of unquestionable
an unquestionable help in carrying out this work.
Please accept the expression of our deepest gratitude and respect
our greatest respect

To our master and thesis director
Dr Khédija SOUMER
Department of Cardiovascular Surgery
CHU Abderrahmen Mami

I am grateful for the honour you have conferred on me by agreeing
to direct me in this work
I would like to express my infinite gratitude for all the efforts so generously
efforts so generously made to bring this work to fruition.
work
I would like to thank you for your availability, patience, frankness and
and your sympathy throughout the realisation of this work.
work
I have the honour of benefiting from your advice, your attentiveness and your
kindness
I would like to take this opportunity to express my gratitude
and my deep respect

1 INTRODUCTION

Moderate to severe tricuspid insufficiency (TFI) is a common condition, observed in 0.55% of the general population, with a clear predominance of women [1]. Its prevalence increases with age, affecting 4% of patients aged 75 or over, and is comparable to that of aortic stenosis or mitral insufficiency [1].

The mechanism of IT is functional in 90% of cases, following dilatation of the right atrium (RA) and tricuspid annulus (TA) and/or remodelling of the right ventricle (RV) [1,2]. This functional tricuspid leak is often associated with left heart valve disease, in around 50% of cases [1,3], but it can also develop late after left valve surgery (mitral and/or aortic) [4,5].

For several years, the tricuspid leak concomitant with left heart valve disease(s) was not repaired, due to the prevailing theory that it improves after valve surgery [6]. However, long-term results have not supported this hypothesis and have shown that after surgical correction of left-sided valve disease, TIA may progressively decrease, remain stationary or continue to evolve and worsen [6,7].

The latter situation, where TIA becomes significant after left-sided valve repair, has recently been reported in a number of articles, underlining the importance of this complex problem in recent decades [4,5]. Studies indicate that late TIA life expectancy and that re-operation for these patients is associated with high short- and long-term morbidity and mortality [8].

According to the latest recommendations from the ESC [2] and the AHA/ACC [9], the surgical indications for CHF are based primarily on the severity of the condition and the size of the annulus. Therefore, patients with moderate to severe CHF should have tricuspid valve repair concomitant left heart surgery. In other cases, repair may be considered in patients with minimal to moderate TIA with a dilated tricuspid annulus (> 40 mm or> 21 mm/m^2) and proposed for left-sided valve surgery. However, the indication remains controversial in a large number of patients with an initially minimal to moderate TIA whose subsequent evolution is unknown. It is therefore essential to identify these patients who are at risk of worsening their CHF and who are candidates for repeat surgery after correction of their left heart valve disease.

In this work, we present a series of patients who underwent left heart valve surgery with minimal to moderate tricuspid insufficiency deemed non-surgical preoperatively and intraoperatively at the cardiovascular surgery centre at the Abderrahmen Mami Hospital.

The objectives our study were to :

- To study the evolution of minimal to moderate unrepaired tricuspid insufficiency after left heart surgery (mitral and/or aortic valve replacement).

- To identify factors associated with worsening of tricuspid leakage after left heart valve surgery.

2 METHODS

1. Type, location and period of study :

This is a retrospective, monocentric, descriptive, longitudinal study conducted in the cardiovascular surgery department of the Abderrahmane Mami University Hospital in Ariana, between January 2018 and December 2022.

2. Study population :

2.1. Inclusion criteria :

We included in the study all patients operated on for left heart valve disease(s) associated with minimal to moderate tricuspid leakage that was not deemed surgical preoperatively and intraoperatively.

- Left heart valve surgery was performed on patients who had either :
- An isolated procedure on the mitral valve involving mitral plasty or valve replacement with a mechanical prosthesis or bioprosthesis.
- An isolated procedure on the aortic valve involving valve replacement with a mechanical prosthesis or bioprosthesis.
- A procedure on both the mitral and aortic valves.

- A minimal to moderate tricuspid leak judged by ultrasound to be non-surgical, whether or not associated with :

- Preoperative :

A tricuspid annulus> 35 mm and < 40 mm

Pulmonary arterial hypertension (PAH) > 40 mmHg

A dilated left atrium (SOG> $20cm^2$)

Dilated right cavities

- Intra-operative findings which ruled out the indication for a procedure on the tricuspid valve. These findings were based on the absence of dilatation of the right cavities and a satisfactory "water test" showing good coaptation of the tricuspid valve leaflets.

2.2. Non-inclusion criteria :

Not included:

- Patients who have undergone tricuspid valve surgery associated with left-sided valve surgery
- Patients who have had ascending aortic surgery associated with left valve surgery
- Patients who have had coronary surgery associated with left valve surgery

The last two groups were not included so as not to bias the factors associated with worsening of tricuspid damage after left heart valve surgery .

2.3. Exclusion criteria :

The following were excluded:

- Patients who cannot be reached by telephone.
- Patients with incomplete medical records: lack of observation notebook, intra-operative data or post-operative follow-up.

3. Aims of the study :

- To study the evolution of minimal to moderate unrepaired tricuspid insufficiency after left heart surgery.
- To identify factors associated with worsening of tricuspid leakage after left heart valve surgery.

4. Conduct of the study :

Epidemiological and clinical data were collected from medical records according to a pre-established data processing form specifying several variables extracted from these records (Appendix 1). This included :

4.1. Epidemiological characteristics :

Age at admission, gender, weight and height determining body mass index (BMI), cardiovascular risk factors including diabetes, hypertension, smoking, dyslipidaemia and Euroscore II were recorded.

The Euroscore II or European System for Cardiac Operative Risk Evaluation predicts mortality by calculating the probability of perioperative death [10].

4.2. Factors linked to the terrain

We identified factors related to the patient's condition that could modify the perioperative context. These factors were divided into three groups:

4.2.1. Medical history

We noted :

- The presence of other concomitant pathologies such as a cerebrovascular accident (CVA), chronic bronchopneumopathy (COPD), chronic renal insufficiency (CRF) or dysthyroidism.
- Taking anticoagulants or platelet aggregation inhibitors. These drugs were stopped 5 days before the operation in order to minimise the risk of bleeding during and after the operation.

4.2.2. Factors linked to valvulopathy

We noted :

- A history of rheumatic fever (RF)
- History of percutaneous mitral dilatation (PMDD)
- The context of infectious endocarditis
- A history of cardiac surgery such as mitral or aortic valve replacement.

4.2.3. Factors that may influence the surgical procedure

An emergency situation and a delay in surgery compared with the diagnosis of valvulopathy could make the operation more difficult.

4.3. Pre-operative patient assessment

4.3.1. Clinical data

Patients were admitted to hospital on an outpatient or emergency basis. They were initially seen and monitored in cardiology departments or by free-lance cardiologists.

All patients were assessed for functional impairment, in particular dyspnoea classified according to NYHA (Appendix 2) with or without other symptoms such as chest pain, syncope and equivalent, signs of right and/or left heart failure, fever, palpitations and embolic events.

4.3.2. Paraclinical data

All patients had :

- An electrocardiogram to look for rhythm disorders such as flutter or atrial fibrillation (AF), and conduction disorders.
- A pre-operative biological work-up and a frontal chest X-ray to analyse the cardiac silhouette and detect pulmonary overload.
- An ETT studying the following parameters:

Assessment of left ventricular ejection fraction (LVEF): According to US guidelines, a normal LVEF varies between 53% and 73% (52-72% for men, 5474% for women). A dysfunction is said to be minimal if the LVEF is between 41% and 52%. Moderate LV dysfunction is defined as between 30% and 40%. Severe dysfunction is defined as a LVEF of less than 30% [11].

Assessment of LV diameters: According to the recommendations of the American Society of Echocardiography (ASE), a normal LV end-diastolic diameter (LVEDD) ranges from 37.8-52.2 mm for women and 42-58.4 mm for men [11].

Impact on the heart chambers, in particular left ventricular hypertrophy/dilatation

Estimation of the surface area of the left atrium (LA): The size of the LA is measured at the end of ventricular systole when its dimensions are at their maximum. The normal surface area of the LV is less than 20 cm^2 [11].

Estimation of right atrial (RA) volume: The size of the DO should be measured at the end of ventricular systole, when the DO chamber is at its largest, before opening of the tricuspid valve [12]. Normal DO volume ranges from 25 ± 7 m/m2 in men to 21 ± 6 ml/m2 in women [11].

Estimation of the function and size of the VD :

TAPSE: TAPSE should be used routinely as a simple method of estimating LV function [12]. A reference value of less than 17 mm indicates right ventricular dysfunction [11].

S': Measuring S' using pulsed tissue Doppler is a simple and reproducible method of assessing LV free wall function [12]. An S' < 9.5 cm/s indicates LV dysfunction [11].

Shortening fraction (SF): The two-dimensional study of the RF is one of the methods of quantitative estimation of the function of the VD [12]. A value of <35% indicates LV dysfunction [11].

Pulmonary arterial pressures: These are considered high when they exceed 35 mmHg [12]. Pulmonary arterial hypertension (PAH) is said to be severe when it exceeds 55 mmHg.

Assessment of tricuspid involvement :

The grade of the leak: the integration of several ultrasound parameters is necessary to determine the grade of the leak. The leak may be minimal, moderate or severe [2,13].

Table I summarises the ultrasound criteria used to assess the degree of IT.

Table I: Ultrasound parameters used to assess tricuspid insufficiency

	Minime	**Moderate**	**Severe**
SOR (cm^2)	< 0.2	0.2-0.4	>0.4
VR (ml)	< 30	30-44	> 45
VC (cm)	< 0.3	0.3 - 0.69	> 0.7

SOR: Surface area of regurgitant orifice; VR: Volume regurgitated; VC: Vena contracta

The size of the annulus: Significant annular dilatation is defined by an end-diastolic diameter of 40 mm or > 21 mm/m2 in the four-chamber transthoracic slice [13].

Involvement of the mitral and/or aortic valves with quantification of the degree of stenosis or leakage [2,13,14].

- Transoesophageal echocardiography (TEE) to detect the presence of vegetation, abscesses or thrombi. During follow-up of patients undergoing valve replacement surgery, TEE is useful studying the haemodynamic profile of the prosthesis.

- Pre-operative coronary angiography was requested in men over 45, post-menopausal women and patients with other cardiovascular risk factors, in order to detect an associated coronary lesion. An ultrasound of the supra-aortic trunks (EDTSA) was also performed to identify any carotid stenosis.

4.3.3. Anaesthetic evaluation

All patients were assessed by an anaesthetist preoperatively. Anaesthetic risk was assessed using the Physical Status Score (ASA) based on a scale of 1 to 5 (Appendix 3).

4.4. Operating data :

4.4.1. Monitoring and settling the patient :

The patient was monitored intra- and post-operatively by measuring blood pressure, heart rate, o2 saturation, diuresis by bladder catheterisation, core temperature, finger-stick blood glucose, instantaneous electrocardiogram, respiratory monitoring and biological monitoring by blood gas, blood ionogram, blood count, ACT (activated clothing time) and lactate measurement. The operation was performed under general anaesthetic, in the supine position, with the legs together and the arms at the side of the body. The surgeon was positioned on the patient's right and his assistant on the opposite side.

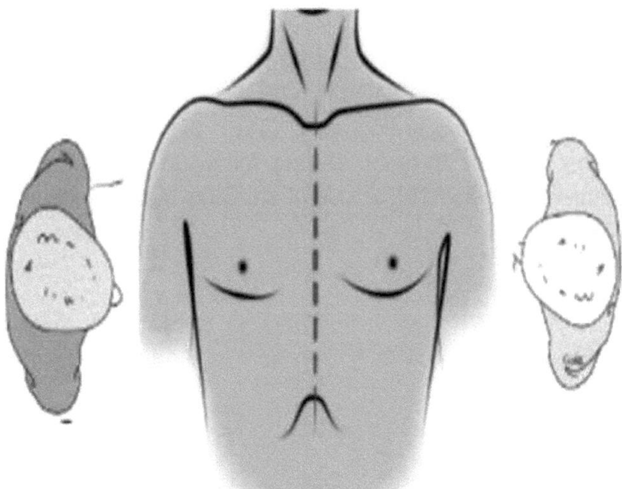

Figure 1: Installation of the patient [15]

4.4.2. Vertical median sternotomy approach:

Vertical median sternotomy is the preferred approach in cardiac surgery. It involves opening the sternum vertically through the middle , giving easy access to the heart and major vessels. It provides adequate exposure for rapid placement of the bypass graft and valve replacement surgery under optimum conditions.

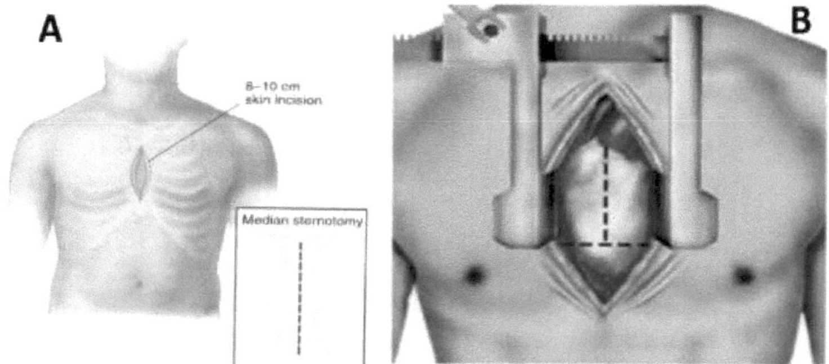

Figure 2: Vertical median sternotomy [15,16].

A. Sternotomy incision

B. Exposure of the heart after sternotomy

4.4.3. Conduct of the CEC :

All valve procedures were performed under extracorporeal circulation (ECG). After systemic heparinisation with 3 mg/Kg sodium heparin and effective anticoagulation, the bypass graft was placed between the ascending aorta and the OD.

Aortic cannulation was performed flush with the brachiocephalic arterial trunk. Venous cannulation was performed through a bursa on the lateral wall of the os via a monocannula in the case of aortic valve replacement or a double superior and inferior vena cava cannulation in the case of mitral or mitro-aortic valve surgery (Figure 3).

LV unloading was ensured by cannulation of the right superior pulmonary vein in the case of aortic valve replacement and by trans-OG unloading in the case of mitral surgery. Arrest of the heart was ensured by a cardioplegia solution, in normothermia, passed through the root of the aorta or selectively via the coronary ostia, at the time of aortic clamping.

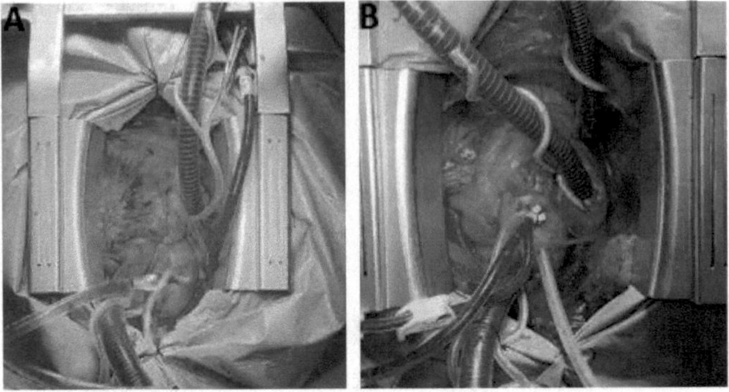

Figure 3: Surgical view of an installed extracorporeal circulation
A. Aorto-caval extracorporeal circulation
B. Aorto-bicaval extracorporeal circulation

4.4.4. Approach to the left heart :

4.4.4.1. Aortic valve approach :

The trans-aortic route is the preferred route for accessing the aortic valve. After aortic clamping, a transverse or oblique aortotomy is performed on the anterior surface of the aorta. The incision is extended upwards on the left towards the pulmonary artery, and downwards on the right towards the middle of the non-coronary sinus.

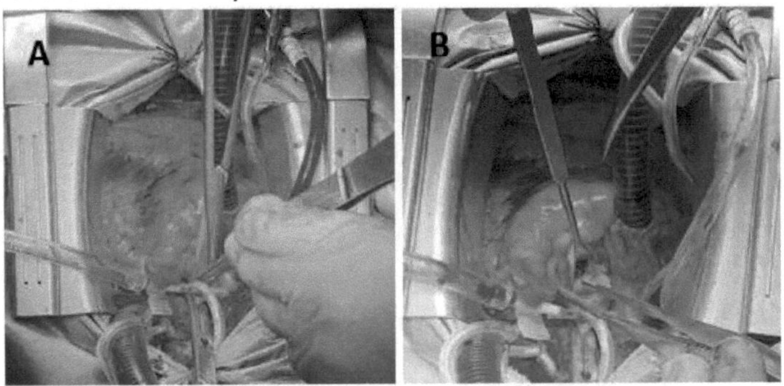

Figure 4: Intraoperative view of a transverse aortotomy
A. Incision of the aorta B. Aortotomy exposing the valve

4.4.4.2. Approach to the mitral valve :

All patients undergoing mitral surgery had a left atriotomy. The incision was made in the right superior vein behind Sondergaard's sulcus. The incision was then extended upwards and downwards.

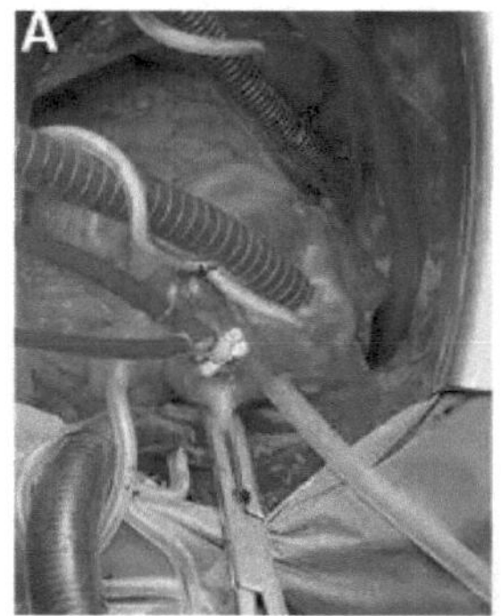
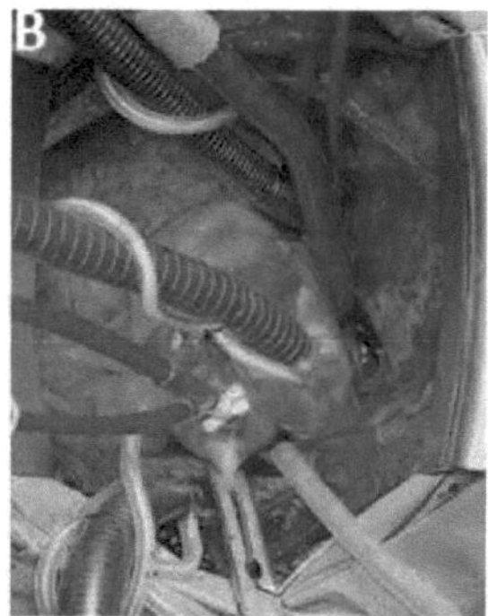
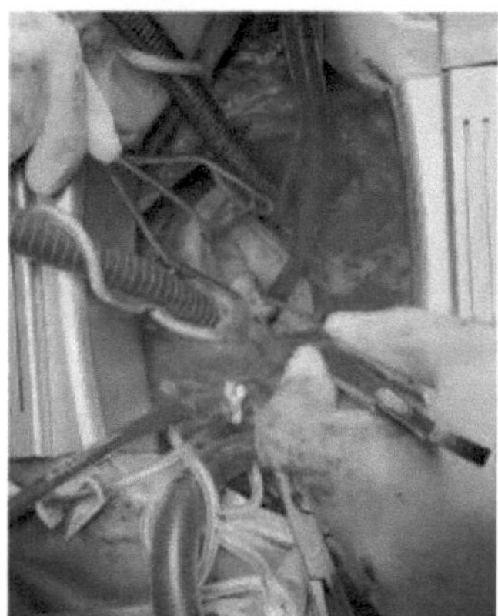

Figure 5: Left atriotomy

A- Left auricle incised behind Sondergaard's sulcus

B- Widening the incision

C- Exposure of the mitral valve after placement of the retractor

4.4.5. Valvular gesture :

4.4.5.1. Mitral plasty :

Patients with valvular or subvalvular changes suitable for conservative surgery underwent mitral plasty to restore normal valve function. The techniques used were :

- Quadrangular resection of the posterior leaflet combined with a sliding plasty: In this case, the valve tissue where the prolapse is located is resected and removed from the annulus, then reinserted by sliding the two valve segments together to suture them edge to edge.
- Triangular resection of the posterior leaflet: The valve tissue containing the lesion is resected in a triangular shape, then sutured directly with separate stitches.
- Open heart mitral commissurotomy (OCMC): We proceeded by incising the fused commissure(s) from towards the free edge and after locating the superior subvalvular apparatus.

All these procedures completed by mitral annuloplasty using a semi-rigid Carpentier annulus to stabilise the native annulus.

4.4.5.2. Mitral valve replacement (MVR) :

After left atriotomy, the anterior leaflet of the mitral valve was resected close to the annulus, taking its main cords with it, while the posterior leaflet was preserved in the absence of calcification, in order to prevent post-operative LV dysfunction.

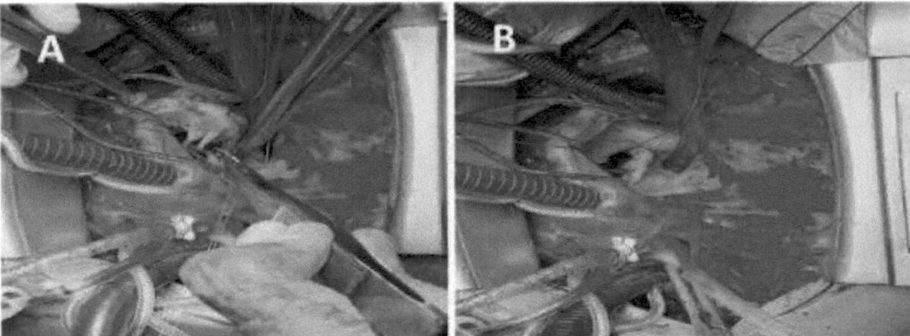

Figure 6: Mitral valve resection

A: Resection of the large mitral valve

B : Conservation and plication of the small mitral valve

Once the valve has been resected, sizing of the ring is ensured by

using a measuring device. All patients who had undergone mitral valve replacement were fitted with intra-annular U-stitches.

When fitting the prosthesis, the anatomical relationships of the mitral valve with the aortic valve, the conduction pathways and the circumflex artery were taken into account.

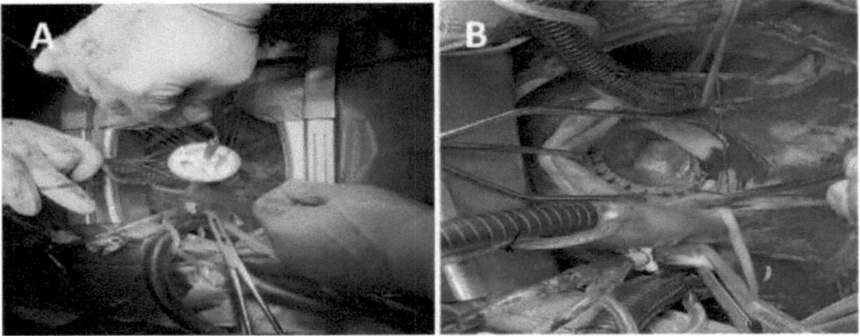

Figure 7: Intraoperative view of mitral valve replacement with a bioprosthesis

A. Fixation of the mitral bioprosthesis using U-stitches

B. Mitral bioprosthesis in place

4.4.5.3. Aortic valve replacement :

After aortotomy, resection of the aortic sigmoid was carried out delicately to avoid disseminating friable calcareous or septic debris into the aorta, LV or coronary arteries. The diameter of the ring was measured by a tester to select the appropriate size of prosthesis. The prosthesis was fixed in the intra-annular position using either U-shaped stitches, three overjections or simple stitches.

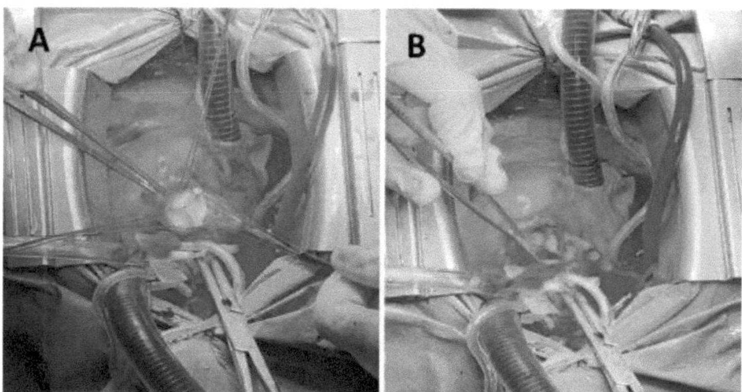

Figure 8: Intraoperative view of aortic valve replacement with bioprosthesis
A. Fixation of the bioprosthesis using U points
B. Fitting the bioprosthesis

4.4.6. Redux surgery of the tricuspid valve :

After left heart surgery, some patients in our series had worsened their initial tricuspid lesions, which were quantified as minimal to moderate, and required repeat surgery.

These patients underwent either a conservative procedure on the tricuspid valve or a replacement of the latter, with or without a procedure on the mitral and/or aortic valve or prosthesis.

4.4.6.1. Approach :

All patients undergoing tricuspid valve surgery were approached via a right atriotomy. The incision was made parallel to the right atrioventricular groove and extending from the atrium towards the inferior vena cava.

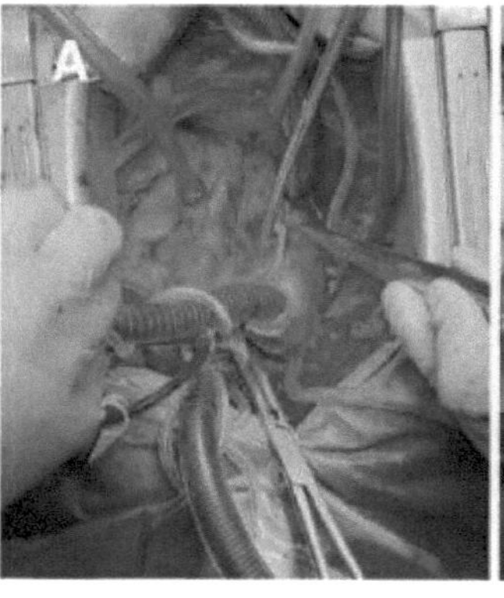

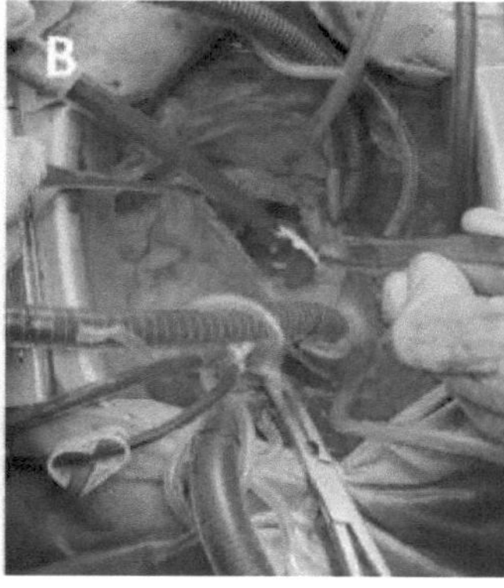

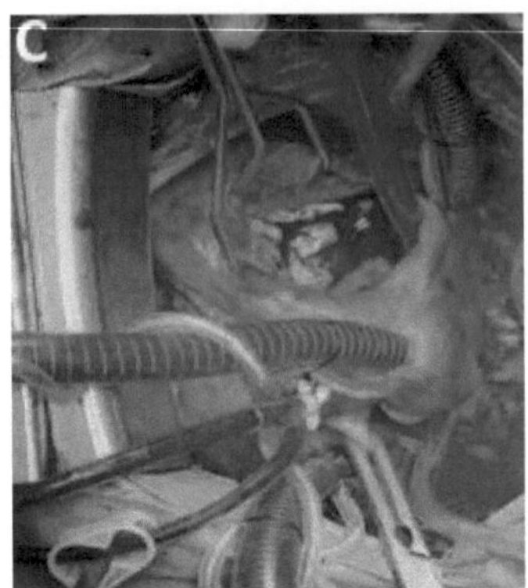

Figure 9: Surgical view of a right auriculotomy

A. Incision of the right atrium

B. Right auricolotomy extended to the inferior vena cava

C. Exposure of the tricuspid valve

4.4.6.2. Action on the tricuspid valve :

- Tricuspid annuloplasty :

Once the tricuspid valve had been exposed, the condition of its leaflets was checked to ensure that the conservative procedure was indicated. In such situations, tricuspid annuloplasty was performed using a Carpentier ring fixed with U-shaped stitches, while respecting the area of conduction tissue.

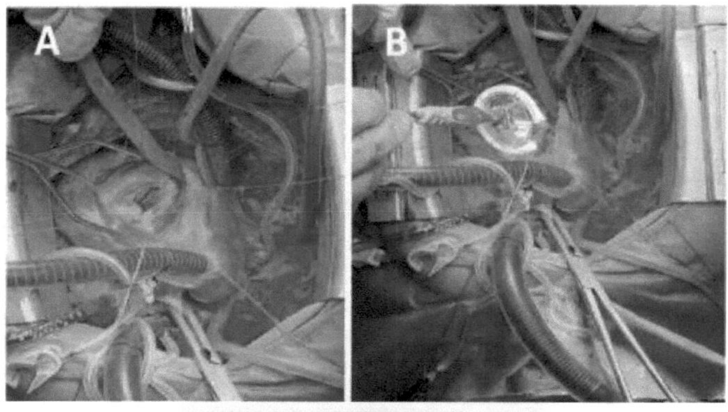

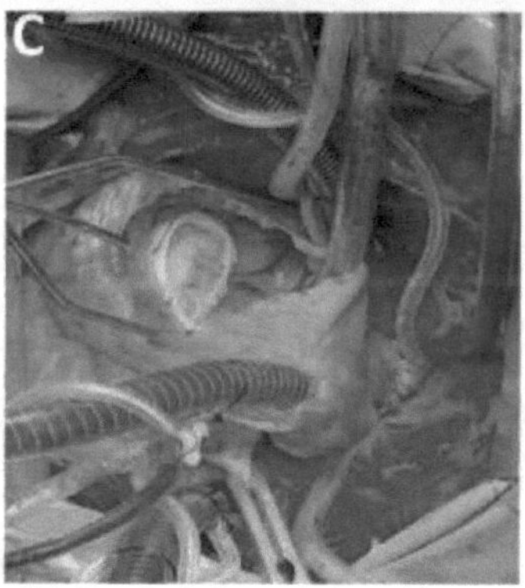

Figure 10: Surgical view of tricuspid annuloplasty

A. Exposure of the tricuspid valve

B. Fixation of the ring by U-shaped points sparing the zone of passage of the conduction pathways

C. Placement of the tricuspid annulus

- Tricuspid valve replacement :

In patients with significant valve lesions, the tricuspid valve was replaced by a bioprosthesis.

The bioprosthesis was attached using the remnants of the valve, while respecting the anteroseptal commissure and the anterior part of the inner leaflet.

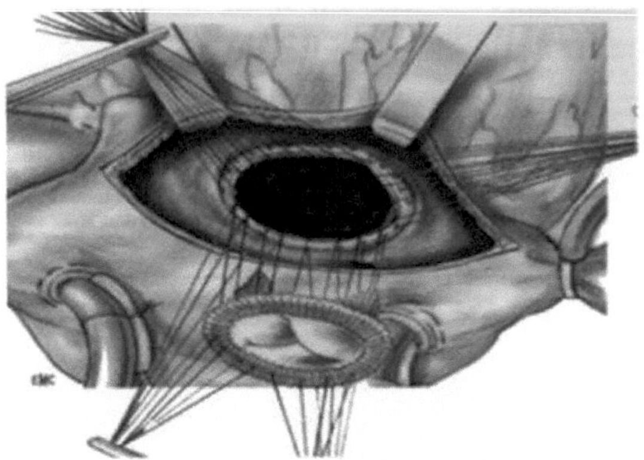

Figure 11: Tricuspid valve replacement by bioprosthesis [17].

4.5. Post-operative course :

4.5.1. Immediate post-operative :

4.5.1.1. Conditioning in intensive care unit :

On leaving the operating theatre, all patients were transferred to a cardiac surgery intensive care unit. Hourly monitoring was based :

- Haemodynamic status: blood pressure, heart rate, electrocardiogram and diuresis.
- The drainage system: We carried out the usual hourly monitoring of suction systems to detect any bleeding.
- Respiratory status: Blood gas measurements were taken regularly to adjust ventilator parameters prior to extubation.
- Sepsis: All patients were given antibiotic prophylaxis with a 1st generation cephalosporin for 48 hours, with monitoring of the thermal profile.
- Biology: A blood test including a blood count, haemostasis test, blood ionogram, renal function test and lactate assay taken at H0 and H06.

We also noted :

- Length of stay in the intensive care unit
- Length of hospital stay
- In-hospital mortality (intra-operative and immediate post-operative)
- Complications arising during resuscitation, such as tamponade, infectious pneumonia, renal failure, stroke, rhythm or conduction disorders, etc.

4.5.1.2. Anticoagulation :

During the first few hours, and in the absence of bleeding, all patients were started on a platelet anti-aggregant based on low-dose acetylsalicylic acid , in accordance with the department's protocol. Anticoagulant treatment was introduced according to the type and position of the implanted prosthesis:
Mechanical prostheses: From H06 onwards, and in the absence of bleeding,

patients who had undergone valve replacement with this type of prosthesis were started on unfractionated heparin (UFH) adjusted by the APTT, then switched to anti-vitamin K (AVK) as soon as the drains were removed.
Bioprostheses: Anticoagulation of patients with bioprostheses in the aortic position was limited to platelet anti-aggregation with acetylsalicylic acid for a period of 3 months.
For bioprostheses in the mitral position, curative anticoagulation was instituted for three months. This anticoagulation was provided by UFH, followed by anti-vitamin K.

4.5.2. Remote post-operative follow-up :

We recorded the short-, medium- and long-term follow-up of patients. Patients were reviewed daily, during their hospital stay and then at the outpatient clinic at one month, 3 months, 6 months and 1 year.
All patients in our series were called and referred to the hospital's cardiology department for clinical and ultrasound assessment.

4.5.2.1. Clinical evaluation :

Clinical examination of the patients revealed :
- Recurrence of dyspnoea and its NYHA stage
- Chest pain
- The notion of syncopation or equivalent
- The concept of palpitations
- The onset of right or left heart failure

4.5.2.2. Ultrasound evaluation :

All patients underwent ultrasound monitoring in the cardiology department of the Abderrahmen Mami Hospital. The objectives of remote postoperative ultrasound were to assess tricuspid leakage after left heart valve surgery and to study the haemodynamic profile of the prostheses.
The various parameters detected by ultrasound were :
- An assessment of the FeVG
- An assessment of LV diameters
- An estimate of the surface area of the OG
- An estimate of the surface area of the DO
- Estimation of the function and size of the VD by measuring TAPSE, S' and FR
- Measurement of pulmonary arterial pressures to look for PAH
- Assessment of tricuspid leakage by estimating the degree of leakage and the size of the annulus.
- An assessment of the haemodynamic profile of the prosthesis(es) in mitral and/or aortic position in search of thrombosis or stenosis or a paraprosthetic leak.

4.5.2.3. Follow-up of re-operated patients :

After the second surgery for worsening tricuspid involvement, patients were contacted for clinical and ultrasound evaluation.

5. Statistical analysis :

The data were entered using Microsoft Office 2016 Excel and analysed using SPSS version 25.0 statistical software.

- Descriptive study :

Qualitative variables were described in terms of observed numbers and frequencies (%).

For quantitative variables, the data distribution was studied using skewness and kurtosis coefficients and normality tests. This study was based on the calculation of means and standard deviations in the case of a normal distribution, and medians and interquartile ranges in the opposite case.

- For the analysis of the association between two qualitative variables, the comparison of two frequencies on independent series was carried out by "Pearson's Chi2 test" in the case of verified conditions of application, and by Fischer's test in the case of non-validity.

- To analyse the association between a qualitative variable and a quantitative variable, two means were compared using the Student's t test in the case of a normal distribution and the non-parametric Mann Whitney test in the opposite case.

- Multivariate analysis was performed using a bivariate logistic regression model (selection threshold p = 0.2). The risk estimate was calculated as the odds ratio (OR) with a 95% confidence interval (95% CI).

We used the significance threshold for p< 5%.

6. Bibliographic research :

Bibliographic research in French and English was carried out using the search engines "scholar.google.com", " www.sciencedirect.com " and " www.ncbi.nlm.nih.gov/pubmed " using the following keywords:

In French: Remplacement valvulaire cardiaque, Insuffisance tricuspide, insuffisance cardiaque droite, oreillette gauche, facteurs associés, évolution, fibrillation auriculaire.

Cardiac valve replacement, tricuspid regurgitation, right heart failure, left atrium, related factors, course, atrial fibrillation.

Zotero" software was used to insert the bibliography.

7. Declarations of interest :

We declare, author and supervisor, that we have no conflicts of interest in relation to this work. None of us, or any of the patients in the series, has been paid or funded by any pharmaceutical industry.

8. Ethical considerations :

Patients called for follow-up were informed of the purpose of our study and gave oral consent for the use of personal data from their medical records.

Personal data was collected with strict respect for patients' anonymity and the confidentiality of their information.

3 RESULTS

1 .DESCRIPTIVE STUDY :

1.1. General information :

Between January 2018 and December 2022, 57 patients had mitral and/or aortic valve replacement with minimal to moderate tricuspid leakage not deemed surgical in the Cardiovascular Surgery Department of Abderrahmen Mami Hospital. 168 patients were not included and 11 were excluded.

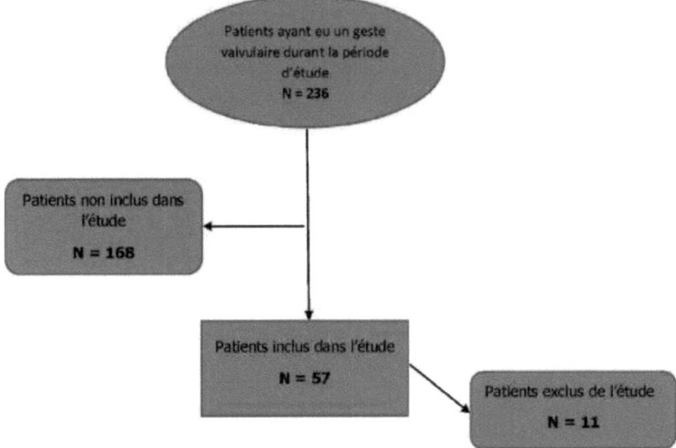

1.2. Demographic characteristics of the study population :

1.2.1. Age :

The average age of the patients was 50.2 years (± 13.9) with extremes ranging from 17 to 82 years (Figure 12).

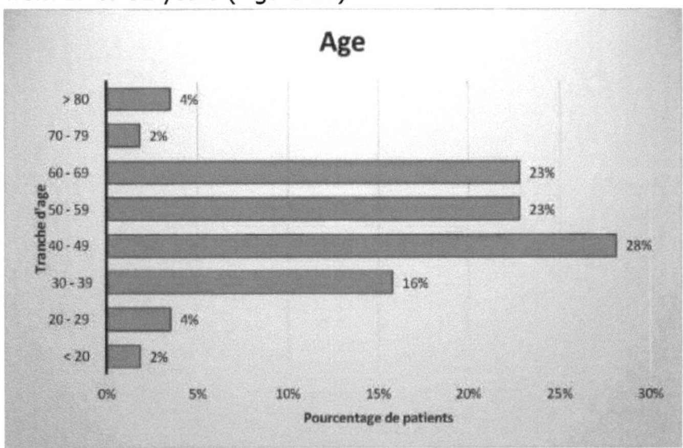

Figure 12: Breakdown of patients by age group

1.2.2. Genre :

Our series of studies showed a clear predominance of females, with a sex ratio of 0.59 (Figure 13).

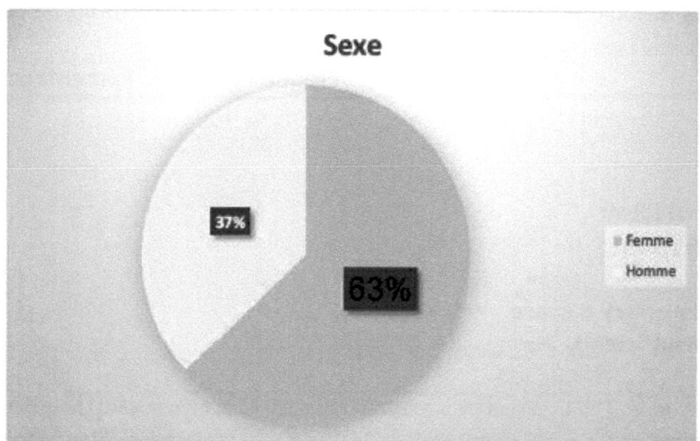

Figure 13: Breakdown of patients by gender

1.2.3. Body mass index (BMI) :

The mean BMI was 26.5 ± 5 kg/m^2 [17.35 - 40.7]. Calculation of BMI showed that 13 subjects were obese (23%) and 18 were overweight (32%).

The table below summarises the anthropometric data.

Table II: Summary of anthropometric measurements

	Average	**Extreme**
Weight (kg)	70,4 ± 11,52	50-103
Height (cm)	163,59 ± 7,68	150-180
BMI (kg/m^2)	26,53 ± 5	17,35-40,7

1.2.4. Cardiovascular risk factors (CVRF) :

The main cardiovascular risk factors studied in our series were smoking, type II diabetes, hypertension and dyslipidaemia.

Figure 14 shows the distribution of patients according to cardiovascular risk factors.

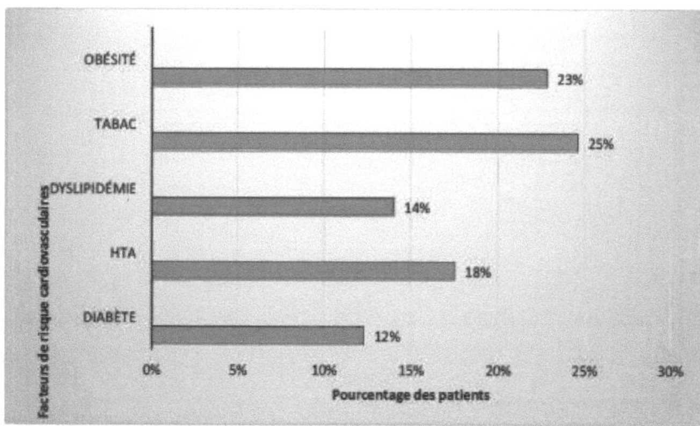

Figure 14: Distribution of patients according to cardiovascular risk factors

1.2.5. Medical history :

The various associated pathologies are summarised in the table below.

Table III: Breakdown of patients by medical history

	Frequency (n)	Percentage (%)
No	6	11
RAA	39	68
DMPC	11	19
Hypothyroidism	5	9
STROKE / TIA	4	7
OSA	3	5
Coronary artery disease	1	2
Renal insufficiency	1	2
COPD	1	2

RAA: rheumatic fever; PMDD: percutaneous mitral dilatation; CVA: cerebrovascular accident; TIA: transient ischaemic attack; OSA: obstructive sleep apnoea syndrome; COPD: chronic obstructive pulmonary disease.

1.2.6. Surgical history :

In the population studied, we observed 7 patients with various surgical histories, but no previous history of cardiac surgery was noted.

1.2.7. Long-term treatment :

A total of 34 patients were on long-term treatment (60%), including 28 on anticoagulants (49%) and 6 on antiplatelet agents (11%).

1.2.8. Etiologies of valvulopathy :

In our series, the main causes of valvulopathy were rheumatic valvulopathy, followed by degenerative pathology, infective endocarditis, Barlow's disease and aortic bicuspidism.

Figure 15 summarises the distribution of patients according to aetiology.

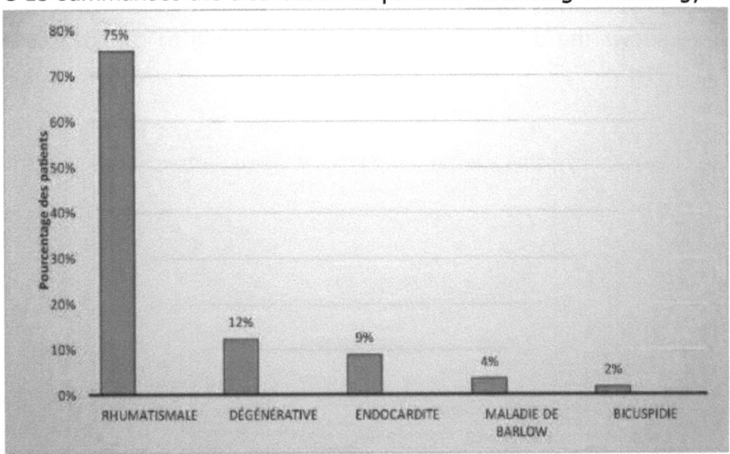

Figure 15: Breakdown of patients by aetiology

1.2.9. Euroscore II :

The mean predicted patient mortality according to Euroscore II was 2.46% ± 1.17 [0.76% - 18.4%].

In our series, 10 patients (18%) had a high risk of mortality with a Euroscore II of more than 5%.

2 .CLINICAL STUDY :

2.1. Functional signs :

The main functional sign was dyspnoea, found in 54 of the patients in our series (95%). Stage III of the NYHA classification was predominant.

The following table summarises the distribution of patients according to the intensity of dyspnoea.

Table IV: Breakdown of patients by NYHA stage

	Frequency (n)	Percentage (%)
Stage I	0	-
Stage II	8	14%
Stage III	34	60%
Stage IV	12	21%

The other reasons for consultation were palpitations and lipothymia, observed in 15 and 13 patients respectively (Figure 16).

Other less frequent signs have led patients to consult a doctor:

- Angina: Nine patients presented with angina chest pain.
- Syncope: A syncopal episode has been reported in three patients.
- Embolic accident: Two patients suffered a cerebrovascular accident .

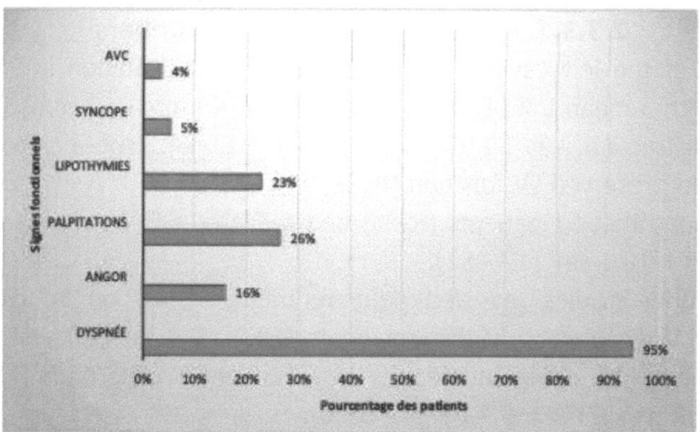

Figure 16: Distribution of patients according to functional signs

2.2. Physical signs :

The physical signs revealed in the subjects in our study were

- An auscultatory abnormality was found at the mitral focus in 42 patients (74%) and at the aortic focus in 15 patients (26%).
- Left, right or congestive heart failure, observed in 6 patients (11%).

- Hemiplegia in 2 patients following a stroke (4%)

2.3. Additional tests:

2.3.1. Electrocardiogram (ECG) :

The ECG was normal in 20 patients (35%). Rhythm disturbances were the most frequent electrical signs.

Table V summarises the electrical signs observed in our patients.

Table V: Distribution of patients according to electrical signs

	Frequency (n)	Percentage (%)
ECG Normal	20	35%
Atrial fibrillation	29	51%
Repolarisation disorders	4	7%
Conduction disorders	9	16%

2.3.2. Chest X-ray :

Chest X-rays were without abnormalities in 11 patients (20%). However, it was pathological in 46 patients (79%).

The table below illustrates the different radiological aspects.

Table VI: Distribution of patients according to radiological aspects

	Frequency (n)	Percentage (%)
Normal	11	19%
Cardiomegaly	40	70%
Mitral silhouette	28	49%
Hilar overload	10	18%

2.3.3. Transthoracic ultrasound (TTE) :

2.3.3.1. Study of the heart chambers :

The study of the left cavities found left ventricular dilatation in 22 patients (38.6%) with a mean LVEDD of 53.6 mm ± 6.5 [40 mm - 67 mm]. The mean LV ejection fraction was 59.9% ± 9.1 [36% - 80%]. In our population, 46 patients had preserved LV function (81%).

We also found that 51 patients (89%) had a dilated OG with a mean OG size of 33.1 cm^2 ± 10.1 cm^2 [17 - 52].

Right chamber studies revealed right ventricular dilatation in five patients (9%) and LV dysfunction in three patients (5%). The mean TAPSE was 21.1 mm ± 2.5 mm [14 - 26], the mean S' was 12.6 cm/s ± 2.3 cm/s [7 - 18] and the mean FR was 53% ± 5.7 [40% - 62%].

We also noted DO dilatation in 30 patients (53%) with a mean DO size of 14.8 cm2 ± 5.6 cm2 [10 - 29].

The pulmonary arterial pressure study concluded that PAH was severe in 12 patients (21%), with a mean of 50.4 mmHg ± 10.8 mmHg [23 mmHg - 80 mmHg].

The table below summarises the ultrasound data for the heart chambers and

LV and VD function.

Table VII: Results of ultrasound parameters of the cardiac cavities

	Frequency (n)	Percentage (%)
VG		
LVEF (%)		
Moderate dysfunction (30%-54%)	11	19
Function retained (> 55%)	46	81
Dilatation of the LV	22	39
LV hypertrophy	17	30
OG expansion	51	89
< 20 cm2	4	7
20 - 40 cm2	39	68
> 40 cm2	14	25
OD expansion	30	53
< 10 cm2	5	9
10-20 cm2	41	72
>20 cm2	11	19
VD		
TAPSE		
> 17 mm	54	95
< 17 mm	3	5
S'		
> 9.5 cm/s	54	95
< 9.5 cm/s	3	5
FR (%)		
VD function retained	54	95
Impaired VD function	3	5
VD dilation	5	9
PAH	53	93
PAPS> 55 mmHg	12	21
PAPS 35-54 mmHg	42	74
PAPS < 35 mmHg	4	7

LV = left ventricle; LVEF = LV ejection fraction; LA = left atrium; RA = right atrium; RV = right ventricle; RF= shortening fraction; PAH = pulmonary arterial hypertension; SBAP= systolic pulmonary artery pressure.

2.3.3.2. Study of valvulopathy :

Mitral valve :

Ultrasound revealed a predominance of mitral valve disease in 49 patients (86%), 32 of whom had isolated mitral disease (56%). Mitral narrowing was found in 35 patients (61%), while mitral insufficiency was observed in 24 others (42%). The mean mitral surface area was 1.2 cm^2 ± 0.28 cm^2 [0.6 - 1.8].

Aortic valve :

Our study included 25 patients with aortic valve disease (44%), 8 of whom had isolated aortic disease (14%). Aortic narrowing was described in 22 patients (39%), while aortic insufficiency was observed in 18 cases (32%). The mean aortic surface area was 0.8 cm2 ± 0.26 cm2 [0.46 - 1.6] and the mean gradient was 51.4 mmHg ± 14.6 [30 - 85].

In our series, 17 patients (30%) had combined mitral and aortic valve disease.

Tricuspid valve :

All patients had minimal to moderate tricuspid insufficiency preoperatively. Of these patients, 19 had minimal TR (33%) and 38 had moderate TR (67%). All patients had an indexed TA < 21 mm/m2 [13.6 - 20.7]. The mean tricuspid annulus size was 31.7 mm ± 2.8 mm [27 - 39]. In our series, 49 patients had a TA < 35 mm (86%), while 8 others had a TA> 35 mm and < 40 mm (14%).

The table below summarises the echographic data for valvulopathy:

Table VIII: Distribution of patients according to echographic data for valvulopathy

	Frequency (n)	Percentage (%)
Isolated mitral valve	32	56
Mitral stenosis	35	61
Mitral insufficiency	24	42
Mitral prolapse	5	9
Mitral surface (SM)		
< 1 cm^2	8	14
1 - 1.49 cm2	23	40
> 1.5 cm2	5	9
Isolated aortic valve	8	14
Aortic stenosis	22	39
Aortic insufficiency Aortic surface area (SAo)	18	32
< 0.5 cm2	1	2
0.5 - 1 cm2	20	35
> 1 cm2	2	4
Medium gradient		
< 40 mmHg	4	7
> 40 mmHg	19	33
Multiple valve surgery: Mitral + Aortic	17	30
Tricuspid valve		
Grade of IT		
Grade 1	19	33
Grade 2	38	67
TA size		
35 mm - 40 mm	8	14
< 35 mm	49	86

2.3.4. Transoesophageal ultrasound (TEE) :

It was performed in five patients in search of intra-uricular thrombus (9%)

and in four patients with infective endocarditis (7%).

2.4. Operating data :

2.4.1. Approach :

All patients were approached by vertical median sternotomy.

2.4.2. Conduct of the CEC :

The average duration of CEC in our patients was 77 ± *21* minutes [37 min - 150 min], while the average duration of aortic clamping was 57 ± 19 minutes [27 min - 124 min].

3 patients (5%) exited the bypass without the need for catecholamines. A total of 49 patients (86%) required low doses of catecholamines at exit from bypass, while five required high doses of vasoactive drugs (9%).

2.4.3. Surgical procedure :

Surgery was performed as an emergency procedure in 11% of cases (6 patients) following complications such as infective endocarditis, embolic events or refractory heart failure.

In our series, mitral valve replacements predominated (74%).

In addition, three patients underwent mitral plasty (5%). This consisted of a quadrangular resection of the posterior leaflet with sliding in one patient, a triangular resection of the posterior leaflet in another and a CMCO in a third.

Figure 17 details the various surgical procedures performed.

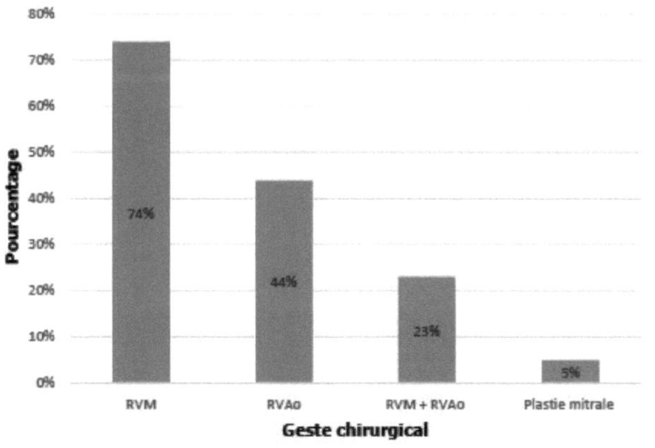

Figure 17: Breakdown of different surgical procedures

2.4.4 Intraoperative complications :

Intraoperative events occurred in 20 patients. Rhythm disturbances were observed in 12 patients (21%), and intraoperative bleeding in a further 12 (21%).

No intraoperative deaths were reported in our series.

2.5. Postoperative data :

2.5.1. Intensive care unit management :

During the ICU stay, the average extubation time was 4 ± 2.5 hours [1h - 24h]. The average length of stay in intensive care was 3 ± 5 days [2 - 9].

Of the patients operated on, 48 were transferred to the intensive care unit on vasoactive drugs (85%). Of these, 46 were easily weaned off catecholamines (81%) and two were difficult (4%).

Transfusion in the intensive care unit was necessary for 29 patients (51%) in different circumstances, either in the context of active postoperative bleeding, or remotely.

Heparin-based curative anticoagulation was used in 51 patients (90%) with a target aPTT of 2.5 - 3.5 times the control. This anticoagulation was used in patients who had undergone valve replacement by mechanical prosthesis , or biological prosthesis in the mitral position, or mitral plasty. On the other hand, six patients were put on preventive anticoagulation, of interest to those who had undergone aortic valve replacement by bioprosthesis.

All patients received antibiotic prophylaxis with a 1st generation cephalosporin for the first 48 hours. Curative antibiotic therapy was required for 35 patients (61%) in the presence of clinical, radiological and biological signs.

2.5.2. Care after transfer to the ward :

After transfer to the cardiovascular surgery department and removal of the drains, patients on curative-dose heparin were started on VKAs.

Total hospital stay was 11 ± 5.2 days [6 - 26].

2.5.3. Postoperative morbidity and mortality :

2.5.3.1. Mortality :

No cases of early mortality were reported in our study series.

2.5.3.2. Morbidity :

Early postoperative complications were observed in 48 patients, representing an overall morbidity of 84%, while nine others had a favourable outcome (16%).

Rhythm disorders :

Atrial fibrillation was the most frequent post-operative complication observed in 31 patients (54%). Two patients who were in sinus rhythm before the operation went into AF post-operatively. The 29 patients who were in AF preoperatively retained this arrhythmia after the operation.

Pulmonary complications :

- **Infectious causes :**

Infectious pneumonitis was the most frequent respiratory complication. It was observed in 51% of patients (29 cases) with a favourable outcome on antibiotic therapy. No patient required reintubation.

- **Acute pulmonary oedema (APO):**

We noted the occurrence of postoperative PAO in 20 patients (35%), related to a hypertensive peak in 12 patients and iterative transfusions in the others. All patients progressed favourably on diuretics and non-invasive ventilation.

Bleeding complications :

Of the 57 patients operated on, seven (12%) experienced post-operative bleeding. Three of these patients presented with tamponade complicated by haemorrhagic shock, requiring urgent revision surgery for 65% of them.

a haemostasis check. In the other four patients, the haemostasis disorders were controlled medically and with blood products. All these patients progressed well after the haemorrhagic episode.

Conductive disorders :

Postoperative conduction problems were noted in two patients (4%), in the form of 3rd degree AVB. In both cases, these conduction problems were transient and did not require the use of a pacemaker.

Neurological complications :

Two cases of post-extubation agitation were described, which regressed spontaneously. This agitation was not accompanied by localisation signs, with normal brain imaging.

Renal complications :

In our series, two patients developed acute renal failure postoperatively (4%), one of whom required haemodiafiltration. Both patients had a favourable outcome, with resumption of diuresis and improvement in clearance.

Parietal infections :

Three of the 57 patients operated on developed a parietal infection of the sternotomy wound, without associated sternal instability (5%). These patients were diabetic, with disturbed postoperative glycaemic figures. All three patients progressed satisfactorily with antibiotic treatment and local care.

Table IX summarises the various postoperative complications.

Table IX: Distribution of patients according to postoperative complications

	Frequency(n)	Percentage (%)
Bleeding complications	7	12
Bleeding without recovery	4	7
Surgical revision	3	5
Pulmonary complications	49	89
Infectious causes	29	51
OAP	20	35
IRA	2	4
FA	31	54
Conduction disorder	2	4
Agitation	2	4
Superficial sternal infection	3	5

OAP = Acute pulmonary oedema, ARF= Acute renal failure, AF= = Atrial fibrillation
Acute acute myocardial infarction.

2.6. Medium- and long-term monitoring :

All patients who survived the hospital stay were contacted and monitored clinically and by echocardiography.

The mean follow-up time between surgery and the last consultation was 42.1 months with extremes ranging from 12 to 67 months.

2.6.1. Late mortality :

Two cases of late death were reported during post-operative follow-up (4%) following heart failure within 12 months in the first case and at 14 months in the second case due to an undetermined cause.

2.6.2. Clinical course :

Of the 55 surviving patients, eight became completely asymptomatic.

Of the 54 patients with dyspnoea preoperatively, we noted a regression of dyspnoea in 12 patients (22%) with persistence of other functional signs, and the 42 others still had dyspnoea. For the latter, an improvement in dyspnoea was observed in 10 patients (24%), who progressed from NHYA stage III to stage II.

Of the patients with preoperative palpitations, seven improved and eight retained them. Three patients had lipothymia remote from the perioperative episode in connection with a stenosing aortic prosthesis, and only one patient reported a postoperative syncopal episode following aortic prosthesis thrombosis.

The table below illustrates the various clinical signs observed postoperatively.

Table X: Breakdown of patients by remote symptomatology

	Frequency (n)	Percentage (%)
Dyspnoea	42	74
NYHA I	3	5
NYHA II	29	51
NYHA III	7	12
NYHAIV	3	5
Syncope	1	2
Lipothymia	3	5
Palpitations	8	14
Chest pain	7	12

2.6.3. Ultrasound evolution :

All surviving patients had an ultrasound examination. The mean follow-up time between surgery and ultrasound examination ranged from nine to 60 months.

The various ultrasound parameters studied were :

2.6.3.1. Study of the left heart :

Postoperative echocardiography of the left cavities showed that 15 of 22 patients retained LV dilatation, with a regression of the mean LVEDD to 51.1 mm ± 6.6 mm [32 - 66]. On the other hand, the mean LVEF fell slightly postoperatively to 56.2% ± 7.4% compared with 59.9% ± 9.1 preoperatively, with LVEF retained in 41 patients (75%).

For the OG, we noted that all patients with dilatation of the OG preoperatively retained it after surgery (51 patients) with a reduction in the mean size of the OG compared with preoperatively, to 31 cm^2 ± 9.3 cm^2 [14.7 - 56.4].

A study of the haemodynamic profile of the mitral prosthesis found that five patients had moderately stenosing prostheses (9%) that were clinically asymptomatic, while three others had minimal para-prosthetic leakage (5%). Only one case of prosthesis thrombosis was described (2%).

Of the 25 patients operated on for aortic valve replacement, four developed a para-prosthetic leak postoperatively, which was considered minimal (7%), and two others had a moderately stenosing prosthesis (4%). Only one patient had a thrombosis of the prosthesis in the aortic position (2%).

Table XI shows the postoperative ultrasound data for the heart chambers and LV and VD function.

Table XI: Ultrasound data of the left creur postoperatively

	Frequency (n)	Percentage (%)
Left ventricle (LV)		
LVEF		
30 - 54 %	14	26
> 55%	41	75
LV dilation	15	27
HVG	16	29
Left auricle (OG)		
OG expansion	51	93
< 20 cm^2	4	7
20 - 40 cm2	44	80
> 40 cm2	7	13
Mitral valve		
Prosthesis thrombosis	1	2
Stenotic prosthesis	5	9
Paraprosthetic leak	3	5
Aortic valve		
Prosthesis thrombosis	1	2
Stenotic prosthesis	2	4
Paraprosthetic leak	4	7
Aortic stenosis	1	2
Aortic insufficiency	2	4

LVEF= Left ventricular ejection fraction; LVH= Left ventricular hypertrophy

2.6.3.2. Study of the right heart :

Study of the right cavities revealed postoperative dilatation of the VD in 14 patients (26%), eight of whom had right ventricular dysfunction (15%). The mean TAPSE was 19.5 mm ± 2.8 mm [11 - 26], the mean S' was 11.2 cm/s ± 2 cm/s [6.5 - 15] and the mean FR was 51% ± 6.6% [35% - 65%].

We found postoperative dilatation of the DO in 47 patients (86%), with an increase in size compared with preoperative to 18.4 cm^2 ± 6.7 cm^2 [9 - 41].

We also noted an improvement in mean postoperative pulmonary artery pressures to 41.9 mmHg ± 11.5 [25 mmHg - 80mmHg], although eight patients developed severe postoperative PAH.

A study of the evolution of the TIA postoperatively showed that 15 patients had worsened their TIA (27%). Of these, 10 had moderate to severe IT (18%), while five others had severe IT (9%).

At follow-up, we noted that 35 patients had a TA> 35 mm (64%) postoperatively compared with 8 patients preoperatively.

The indexed tricuspid annulus study found a mean of 19.3 mm ± 5.4 mm, with 35 patients having an indexed TA< 21 mm/mp (64%). Three patients had a borderline indexed TA preoperatively, these retained a stationary postoperative IT.

Only one patient developed tricuspid narrowing, with moderate IT and a dilated annulus.

Table XII summarises the ultrasound data from the valve and prosthesis study:

Table XII: Postoperative ultrasound parameters of the right heart

	Frequency (n)	Percentage (%)
Tricuspid valve		
Tricuspid insufficiency (TDI)	55	100
Grade 1	13	24
Grade 2	27	49
Grade 3	10	18
Grade 4	5	9
TA size		
> 35 mm	35	64
< 35 mm	20	36
Tricuspid narrowing	1	2
Right auricle (RA)		
Dilatation of the DO	47	86
< 10 cm^2	1	2
10 - 20 cm2	36	66
> 20 cm2	18	33
Right ventricle (RV)	30	53
TAPSE		

< 17 mm	8	15
> 17 mm	47	86
S'		
< 9.5 cm/s	7	13
> 9.5 cm/s	48	87
FR (%)		
VD function retained	49	89
Impaired VD function	6	11
VD dilation	14	25
PAH	53	93
PAPS < 35 mmHg	19	35
PAPS 35-54 mmHg	28	51
PAPS> 55 mmHg	8	15

RD = Right atrium; RV = Right ventricle; TTI = Tricuspid insufficiency; RF = Shortening fraction; PAH = Pulmonary arterial hypertension; SBAP= Systolic pulmonary arterial pressure

2.6.4. Management of patients with moderate to severe tricuspid insufficiency at high procedural risk :

The 10 patients with moderate to severe tricuspid insufficiency after left valve surgery (18%), in whom an indication for isolated tricuspid surgery was not given because of the presence of major PAH and/or a failing VD, were put on optimal medical treatment.

2.6.5. Management of patients developing severe tricuspid insufficiency at low procedural risk :

Redux surgery :

During follow-up, five patients required late repeat surgery to repair tricuspid damage (9%), with or without a procedure on the left heart.

Of these five patients, four underwent tricuspid annuloplasty associated with a left-sided valve procedure, either following dysfunction of the mitro-aortic prostheses in one patient, or mitral plasty that became stenotic in a second, or the appearance of new left-sided heart valve disease in the other two.

Only one patient had an isolated procedure on the tricuspid valve after the initial surgery without recourse to further left heart surgery.

The table below summarises the different revision procedures with the initial surgeries of the left creur.

Table XIII: Different revision procedures and time taken for redux surgery in relation to the time taken to perform the procedure.

initial surgery

Patient N°	Initial surgery	Revision operation	Follow-up time
42	RVM + RVAo	$2^{è}$ RVM + $2^{è}$ RVAo + AT	34
55	RVM	RVT	48
40	Mitral plasty	RVM + AT	52
56	RVAo	RVM + AT	55

41	RVM	RVAo + AT	59

MVR = Mitral valve replacement, AVR = Aortic valve replacement, TA= Tricuspid annuloplasty

Postoperative follow-up after recovery :

All re-operated patients had a favourable post-operative course with 100% survival. Dyspnoea regressed in all patients, from NYHA stage III-IV to stage I-II.

Ultrasound monitoring of these patients showed a good haemodynamic profile for the prostheses and a non-stenosing tricuspid annulus.

Table XIV summarises the postoperative evolutionary profile after redux surgery.

Table XIV: Post-operative course of re-operated patients

Post-operative study	
Hospital mortality	0
Intubation time (h)	10,83 ± 4,6
CEC time (min)	85 ± 29
Clamping time	68 ± 33
Circulatory assistance (ECMO)	0
Stay in intensive care	8 ± 3,4
Complications	
Infectious lung disease	1
Conductive disorders	1
IRA	0
Post-operative bleeding	1
Superficial sternal infection	1

ECMO = Extracorporeal membrane oxygenation, ARF= Acute renal failureê

3.ANALYTICAL STUDY :

3.1. Factors associated with worsening of tricuspid insufficiency :

In order to study the factors associated with the progression of tricuspid leakage, we compared the pre-, intra- and post-operative data between the 55 patients who survived at a distance, and according to the worsening of the IT postoperatively.

3.1.1. Epidemiological factors :

Worsening of IT was significantly associated with long-term VKA use (p = 0.005). However, age, sex and BMI were not associated with this worsening.

The table below summarises the epidemiological factors incriminated in the aggravation of postoperative IT.

Table XV: Epidemiological factors associated with worsening of post-operative tricuspid insufficiency

	Grade 3-4 (n=15)	**Grade 1-2 (n= 40)**	**p**	**OR [IC95%]**
Age (years)	46,6 ± 15,9	51,2 ± 12,9	0,271	-
Type				
Men	4 (20%)	16 (80%)	0,36	-

Woman	11 (31%)	24 (69%)		-
Weight (kg)	74,3 ± 12,8	68,9 ± 11	0,138	-
Height (cm)	165,3 ± 7,3	162,9 ± 7,9	0,312	-
BMI (kg/m²)	27,5 ± 5	26,2 ± 5,1	0,418	-
< 18.5 kg/m²	0	1 (100%)	1	-
18.5 - 24.9 kg/m2	5 (23%)	17 (77%)	0,537	-
25 - 29.9 kg/m2	8 (42%)	11 (58%)	0,073	-
> 30 kg/m 2	2 (15%)	11 (85%)	0,477	-
Taking medication	14 (42%)	19 (58%)	**0,002**	-
Aspégic	1 (17%)	5 (83%)	1	-
Sintrom	12 (44%)	15 (56%)	**0,005**	-

3.1.2. Clinical data :

3.1.2.1. Cardiovascular risk factors and medical history :

Worsening TIA after left heart surgery was significantly associated with the presence of two or more CVDRFs with p = 0.03; OR=4.421; CI95%=1.08-18.093.

The following table shows the different CDRFs and medical histories associated with the aggravation of TIA.

Table XVI: Cardiovascular risk factors and various pathologies associated with worsening of postoperative tricuspid insufficiency

	Grade 3-4 (n=15)	Grade 1-2 (n= 40)	p	OR [IC95%]
FDRCV	15 (31%)	34 (69%)	0,173	-
> 2 FDRCV	12 (39%)	19 (61%)	**0,03**	4,421 [1,0818,093]
> 3 FDRCV	4 (40%)	6 (60%)	0,434	-
Diabetes	4 (57%)	3 (43%)	0,079	-
Tobacco	3 (23%)	10 (77%)	1	-
HTA	1 (11%)	8 (89%)	0,417	-
Dyslipidemia	3 (37%)	5 (63%)	0,669	-
Overweight	7 (41%)	10 (59%)	0,189	-
Obesity	2 (15%)	11 (85%)	0,477	-
Medical history	13 (29%)	32 (71%)	0,71	-
RAA	12 (32%)	26 (68%)	0,344	-
DMPC	3 (27%)	8 (73%)	1	-
Hypothyroidism	2 (40%)	3 (60%)	0,606	-
AVC	1 (25%)	3 (75%)	1	-
IRC	0 (0%)	1 (100%)	1	-
Coronary artery disease	0 (0%)	1 (100%)	1	-
OSA	0 (0%)	3 (100%)	0,554	-
COPD	1 (100%)	0 (0%)	0,273	-
Endocarditis	0 (0%)	4 (100%)	0,565	-
Surgical history	2 (29%)	5 (71%)	1	-

CVRDF: Cardiovascular risk factors; ATH: Hypertension; RAA: Rheumatic fever; PMD: Percutaneous mitral dilatation; CVA: Cerebrovascular accident; CKD: Chronic renal failure; OSA: Obstructive sleep apnoea syndrome; COPD: Chronic obstructive pulmonary disease.

3.1.2.2. Etiologies of valvulopathy :

Rheumatic aetiology was more frequently observed in the worsening of postoperative IT (86.6%), although it was not significantly associated with this progression (p = 0.477).

Table XVII illustrates the different aetiologies of valvulopathy associated with progression of IT after left heart surgery.

Table XVII: Etiologies of valvulopathy associated with worsening of tricuspid insufficiency

	Grade 3-4 (n=15)	Grade 1-2 (n=40)	p
Rheumatic	13 (87%)	29 (73%)	0,477
Degenerative	2 (13%)	4 (10%)	0,66
Endocarditis	0 (0%)	5 (13%)	0,308
Bicuspidia	0 (0%)	1 (3%)	1
Barlow's disease	0 (0%)	2 (5%)	1

3.1.2.3. Functional and physical signs :

No clinical factors were associated with worsening of postoperative TIA. On the other hand, progression of IT was observed in all dyspnoeic patients postoperatively, without there being a significant association (p = 0.554).

Furthermore, the presence of AF-type rhythm disorders on the preoperative ECG was significantly associated with worsening of postoperative IT (p=0.001; OR=10.833; CI95%=2.143-54.769).

The following table summarises the clinical data associated with the worsening of IT:

Table XVIII: Post-operative tricuspid associated worsening of insufficiency clinical data

	Grade 3-4 (n=15)	Grade 1-2 (n= 40)	p	OR [IC95%]
Fever	0 (0%)	4 (10%)	0,565	-
Dyspnoea	15 (100%)	37 (93%)	0,554	-
NYHA II	2 (13%)	6 (15%)	1	-
NYHA III	9 (60%)	24 (60%)	1	-
NYHA IV	4 (27%)	7 (18%)	0,468	-
Angina	2 (13%)	6 (15%)	1	-
Left heart failure	2 (13%)	3 (8%)	0,606	-
Lipothymia	5 (33%)	7 (18%)	0,274	-
Syncope	0 (0%)	3 (8%)	0,554	-
Palpitations	4 (27%)	11 (28%)	1	-
Embolic accident	0 (0%)	2 (5%)	1	-
Euroscore	2,46	2,46	0,334	-
Low risk (0-2%)	3 (21%)	11 (79%)	0,734	-
Medium risk (2-5%)	8 (25%)	24 (75%)	0,655	-
High risk (> 5%)	4 (44%)	5 (56%)	0,236	-
ECG abnormalities	14 (39%)	22 (61%)	**0,008**	11,455 [1,372-95,643]
FA	13 (46%)	15 (54%)	**0,001**	10,833 [2,143-54,769]

Disorders of the conduction	2 (22%)	7 (78%)	1	-
Disorders of the repolarisation	2 (50%)	2 (50%)	0,298	-

AF = Atrial Fibrillation

3.1.3. Ultrasound data :

Study of cavities :

We found that preoperative OG dilatation was significantly associated with postoperative tricuspid leak progression (37.83±8.43 vs 31.35±10.4; p=0.036).

Although DO dilatation was present in 11 of the 15 patients who worsened their postoperative tricuspid leak, it was not significantly associated with this progression (p = 0.061). Moderate PAH was observed in 13 patients with moderate to severe postoperative tricuspid leak, but was not significantly associated with worsening of TI after left valve surgery.

The data are summarised in Table XIX.

Table XIX: Different ultrasound parameters associated with worsening of postoperative tricuspid insufficiency

	Grade 3-4 (n=15)	**Grade 1-2 (n= 40)**	**p**	**OR [IC95%]**
Left ventricle (LV)				
LVEF	57,7 ± 9,8	61,5 ± 8,2	0,159	-
30 - 54 %	3 (20%)	6 (15%)	0,692	-
> 55 %	12 (80%)	34 (85%)		-
DTD	53,5 ± 4,6	53,4 ± 7,1	0,935	-
LV dilation	4 (27%)	17 (43%)	0,282	-
HVG	5 (33%)	11 (28%)	0,744	-
Left auricle (OG)				
Size OG (cm^2)	37,8 ± 8,4	31,3 ± 10,4	**0,036**	1,066 [1,002-1,133]
< 20 cm^2	0 (0%)	4 (10%)	0,565	-
20 - 40 cm2	9 (60%)	28 (70%)	0,529	-
> 40 cm2	6 (40%)	8 (20%)	0,169	-
Right auricle (RA)				
Dilatation of the DO	11 (73%)	18 (45%)	0,061	-
OD size (cm2)	16,7 ± 7,6	14 ± 4,7	0,21	-
< 10 cm2	1 (7%)	4 (10%)	1	-
10 - 20 cm2	8 (53%)	31 (78%)	0,102	-
> 20 cm2	6 (40%)	5 (13%)	0,052	-
Right ventricle (RV)				
TAPSE	21,5 ± 2,9	21,2 ± 2,1	0,714	-
< 17 mm	1 (7%)	1 (3%)	0,475	-
> 17 mm	14 (93%)	39 (74%)		-
S'	12,9 ± 2,6	12,7 ± 2	0,724	-
< 9.5 cm/s	1 (7%)	1 (3%)	0,475	-

> 9.5 cm/s	14 (93%)	39 (97%)		-
FR (%)	52,1 ± 5,8	53,9 ± 5,3	0,3	-
Function VD preserved	1 (7%)	1 (3%)	0,475	-
Impaired VD function	14 (93%)	39 (98%)		-
VD dilation	2 (13%)	2 (5%)	0,298	-
PAH	14 (93%)	37 (93%)	1	-
PAPS	48,5 ± 6	50,3 ± 11,5	0,555	-
> 55 mmHg	1 (7%)	9 (23%)	0,255	-
35-54 mmHg	13 (87%)	29 (73%)	0,477	-
< 35 mmHg	1 (7%)	3 (8%)	1	-

LVEF: Left ventricular ejection fraction; PAH: Pulmonary arterial hypertension; PAPS: Pulmonary arterial systolic pressures; DTD: Telesystolic diameter; LVH: Left ventricular hypertrophy; RF: Shortening fraction.

Valve study :

A large postoperative IT was significantly associated with a mitral surface area of less than 1 cm^2 (p = 0.036).

The following table summarises the echographic valve parameters associated with worsening of tricuspid leakage.

Table XX: Valvular ultrasound parameters associated with worsening of tricuspid insufficiency

	Grade 3-4 (n=15)	**Grade 1-2 (n = 40)**	**P**
Mitral valve			
Mitral stenosis	12 (80%)	22 (55%)	0,089
Mitral insufficiency	4 (27%)	20 (50%)	0,12
Mitral prolapse	2 (13%)	3 (8%)	0,606
Isolated mitral disease	9 (60%)	22 (55%)	0,739
Mitral surface (SM)	1,3 ± 0,2	1,1 ± 0,3	0,068
< 1 cm2	0 (0%)	8 (20%)	**0,032**
1 - 1.49 cm2	10 (67%)	12 (30%)	0,139
> 1.5 cm2	2 (13%)	3 (8%)	1
Aortic valve			
Aortic stenosis	5 (33%)	16 (40%)	0,65
Aortic insufficiency	3 (20%)	15 (38%)	0,335
Isolated aortic disease	1 (7%)	6 (15%)	0,66
Aortic surface area (SAo)	0,9 ± 0,4	0,7 ± 0,2	0,3
< 0.5 cm2	0 (0%)	1 (10%)	1
0.5 - 1 cm2	5 (33%)	14 (35%)	1
> 1 cm2	1 (7%)	1 (10%)	0,481
Medium gradient	54,8 ± 18,7	50,8 ± 13,6	0,577
< 40 mmHg	1 (7%)	3 (8%)	1
> 40 mmHg	5 (33%)	13 (33%)	
Multiple valve surgery : Mitral + Aortic	5 (33%)	12 (30%)	1
Tricuspid valve			
Grade of IT	4 (27%)	14 (35%) 26	0,749

Grade 1	11 (73%)	(65%) 31,9 ± 3	0,11
Grade 2	30,9 ± 1,7 0 (0%)	7 (18%)	0,171
AT size (mm)	15 (100%)	33 (83%)	
35 mm - 40 mm			
< 35 mm			
Indexed AT size (mm)	16,8 ± 1,2	19,6 ± 0,8	0.096
< 21 mm/m2	15 (100%)	35 (100%)	
>21mm/m2	0	0	
Associated lesions			
Thrombus	1 (7%)	4 (10%)	1

Vegetation II 0 (0%)4 (10%)0,565

3.1.4. Intraoperative factors :

Of the 15 patients who worsened their IT postoperatively, 13 had had RVM without there being a significant association (p = 0.304).

Table XXI illustrates the different intraoperative factors associated with the occurrence of moderate to severe IT postoperatively.

Table XXI: Intraoperative factors associated with worsening of tricuspid insufficiency

	Grade 3-4 (n=15)	Grade 1-2 (n = 40)	P
Clamping time (min)	57 [45-90,5]	58 [47-74,5]	0,799
CEC time (min)	80 [63,5-114,5]	76 [60-97,5]	0,472
Catecholamines			
Without catecholamines	0 (0%)	3 (100%)	0,554
Low dose	14 (30%)	33 (70%)	0,423
High dose	1 (20%)	4 (80%)	1
Operative gesture			
Mitral valve replacement	13 (32%)	28 (68%)	0,304
Mechanical engineering	13 (36%)	23 (64%)	0,16
Organic	0 (0%)	5 (100%)	
Mitral plasty	1 (33%)	2 (67%)	1
Aortic valve replacement	6 (25%)	18 (75%)	0,739
Mechanical engineering	6 (32%)	13 (68%)	0,28
Organic	0 (0%)	5 (100%)	
Multiple valve surgery: Mitral + Aortic	5 (39%)	8 (61%)	0,31
Intraoperative complications	4 (21%)	15 (79%)	0,452
Bleeding	3 (25%)	9 (75%)	1
Rhythm disorders	2 (18%)	9 (82%)	0,708

3.1.5. Postoperative factors :

Worsening TIA was significantly associated with postoperative atrial fibrillation (n=13; 45%; p=0.002; OR=9.75; CI95%=1.934-49.146).

The table below summarises the postoperative complications associated with the worsening of IT postoperatively.

Table XXII: Post-operative complications of tricuspid insufficiency associated with the aggravation of

	Grade 3-4 (n= 15)	Grade 1-2 (n= 40)	P
Post-operative complications			
Yes	14 (30%)	32 (70%)	0,417
No	1 (11%)	8 (89%)	
Tamponade			
Yes	2 (29%)	5 (71%)	1
No	13 (27%)	35 (73%)	
Takeover			
Yes	1 (33%)	2 (67%)	1
No	14 (27%)	38 (73%)	
Atrial fibrillation			
Yes	13 (45%)	16 (55%)	**0,002**
No	2 (8%)	24 (92%)	
Atrioventricular block			
Yes	2 (100%)	0 (0%)	0,071
No	13 (25%)	40 (76%)	
Acute lung oedema			
Yes	5 (26%)	14 (74%)	0,908
No	10 (28%)	26 (72%)	
Heart failure			
Yes	1 (100%)	0 (0%)	0,273
No	14 (26%)	40 (74%)	
Infectious lung disease			
Yes	8 (28%)	21 (72%)	0,956
No	7 (27%)	19 (73%)	
Acute renal failureê			
Yes	1 (50%)	1 (50%)	0,475
No	14 (26%)	39 (74%)	
Agitation			
Yes	0 (0%)	2 (100%)	1
No	15 (28%)	38 (72%)	
Parietal infection			
YES I 1 (33%) 2 (67%) 1			
No	1 14 (27%)	38 (73%)	
Length of stay in ICU (days)	3 (2-6)	3 (2-9)	0,25
Length of hospital stay (days)	11 (6-26)	11 (6-23)	0,655

3.2. Multivariate study :

We identified the independent factors associated with worsening of IT postoperatively, after adjusting for age, gender and BMI.

The threshold value of the OG above which the risk of severity was significantly associated was determined by the ROC curve with an estimated threshold value corresponding to a better sensitivity of this parameter in predicting the severity of the TIA.

The table below illustrates the different independent factors for worsening IT postoperatively.

Table XXIII: Multivariate study of factors associated with the worsening of postoperative tricuspid insufficiency

	n (%)	P	OR	IC95%
Anticoagulant treatment	14 (42%)	0,008	18,986	2,128-169,379
> **2 FDRCV**	12 (39%)	0,013	9,457	1,611-55,521
Preoperative AF	13 (46%)	0,004	11,496	2,175-60,767
OG size > 33 cm²	10 (42%)	0,049	3,744	1,005-13,951

CVDRF: Cardiovascular risk factors; AF: Atrial fibrillation; LA: Left atrium

3.3. Comparison of pre- and postoperative clinical and ultrasound signs :

3.3.1. Clinical signs :

We noted that dyspnoea regressed in 12 patients postoperatively, leading to a significantly favourable outcome (p = 0.013). Lipothymia disappeared in 11 patients (p = 0.022).

The tables below describe the evolution of the various clinical signs pre- and postoperatively.

Table XXIV: Comparison of pre- and post-operative dyspnoea

		Post-operative dyspnoea		P
		Yes	**No**	
Dyspnoea pre operating	**Yes**	40	12	**0,013**
	No	2	1	

Table XXV: Comparison of the evolution of lipothymia pre- and post-operatively

		Post-operative lipothymia		P
		Yes	**No**	
Lipothymia pre operating	**Yes**	1	11	**0,022**
	No	2	41	

Table XXVI: Comparison of the evolution of syncope pre- and post-operatively

		Post-operative syncope		P
		Yes	**No**	
Pre-syncope operating	**Yes**	0	3	**0,625**
	No	1	51	

Table XXVII: Comparison of the evolution of palpitations pre- and post-operatively

		Post-operative palpitations		P

		Yes	No	
Palpitations pre-operating	**Yes**	3	12	0,143
	No	5	35	

3.3.2. Ultrasound signs :

We observed a significant decrease in all postoperative ultrasound parameters of the cardiac chambers with the exception of the decrease in the size of the OG (p=0.087).

The table below illustrates the variations in ultrasound parameters pre- and postoperatively.

Table XXVIII: Pre- and post-operative profile of the heart chambers

Parameters	**Pre- and post-operative difference**		- p
	Mean ± SD	IC95%	
LVEF (%)	4,3 ± 8,7	[1,951-6,667]	**0,001**
Telesystolic diameter	2,4 ± 7,6	[0,323-4,44]	**0,024**
Size OG (cm^2)	2,1 ± 8,9	[-0,3196-4,5268]	0,087
OD size (cm2)	-3,6 ± 6,2	[-5,3204--1,9887]	**<0,001**
TAPSE (mm)	1,7 ± 3,2	[0,861-2,5753]	**<0,001**
S' (cm/s)	1,6 ± 2,9	[0,794-2,3624]	**<0,001**
Regurgitation fraction (%)	2,4 ± 7,9	[0,268-4,568]	**0,028**
PAPS (mmHg)	7,9 ± 15,4	[3,787-12,14]	**<0,001**

LVEF: Left ventricular ejection fraction; LO: Left atrium; RA: Right atrium; SBAP: Systolic pulmonary artery pressures.

A significant increase in tricuspid annulus size was observed postoperatively (4.8 ± 5.8 mm; p < 0.001).

The two tables below compare the evolution of TA preoperatively and postoperatively.

Table XXIX: Postoperative evolution of the size of the tricuspid annulus

a	**Pre-postoperative difference**		
	Mean ± SD	IC950/0	**p**
AT size (mm)	4,8 ±5,8	[3,197-6,33]	**<0,001**

AT: Tricuspid ring

Table XXX: Comparison of pre- and post-operative tricuspid annulus size

		Post-operative TA		- p
		> **35mm**	**< 35mm**	
AT pre operating	> **35mm and <40 mm**	6	1	_ **<0,001**
	< 35mm	29	19	

AT: Tricuspid ring

4 DISCUSSION

1 .SUMMARY OF THE MAIN RESULTS :

We conducted a single-centre retrospective study, from January 2018 to December 2022, including 57 patients operated on for left heart valve disease (mitral and/or aortic) with minimal to moderate tricuspid insufficiency deemed non-surgical, at the cardiovascular surgery department of the Abderrahmen Mami University Hospital in Ariana.

The mean age of patients in our series was 50.2 ± 13.9 years, with a clear predominance of females, giving a sex ratio of 0.59:1.

The main cardiovascular risk factors studied in our series were arterial hypertension (17%), smoking (25%), dyslipidaemia (14%) and diabetes (12%). The majority of patients had at least two cardiovascular risk factors (37%).

A total of 34 patients were on long-term treatment (60%), including 28 on anticoagulants (49%) and six on antiplatelet agents (11%).

Rheumatic valve disease was the most common aetiology. It was present in 43 patients (75%), followed by degenerative pathology in 7 patients (12%), then infective endocarditis in 5 patients (9%).

The main functional sign was dyspnoea, found in 54 of the patients in our series (95%). Stage III of the NYHA classification was predominant in 34 patients (60%), followed by stage IV in 21%.

Rhythm disorders were the most frequent electrical signs, including 29 patients with complete atrial fibrillation (51%).

A study of the ultrasound parameters found that 51 patients had OG dilatation (89%) with a mean size of 33.1 cm^2 [17 - 52]. Right ventricular dilatation was observed in five patients (9%) and LV dysfunction in a further three (5%). In addition, OD dilatation was observed in 30 patients (53%) with a mean size of 14.8 cm2 [10 - 29]. Severe PAH was observed in 12 patients (21%) with a mean of 50.4 mmHg [23-80].

The valvular study showed that mitral valve involvement was predominant, present in 49 patients (86%). Aortic involvement was observed in 25 cases (44%).

All patients had minimal to moderate tricuspid insufficiency preoperatively with an indexed TA < 21 mm/m2, of which 49 had a TA < 35 mm (86%), while a further 8 had a TA> 35 mm and <40 mm (14%).

All patients were operated on under CEC with aortic clamping. Mitral valve replacement was performed in 42 patients (74%), while aortic valve replacement was performed in 25 patients (44%).

Early postoperative complications were observed in 48 patients, giving an overall morbidity of 84%. Two patients, who were in sinus rhythm before the operation, went into AF post-operatively, and two others presented a conductive disorder such as transient 3rd degree AVB (3%).

The average length of stay in intensive care was 3 days [2-9]. The total length hospital stay was 11 days [6-26].

No cases of peri-operative mortality were reported in our study.

All patients contacted for post-operative follow-up. The mean follow-up time between surgery and the last consultation was 42.1 months.

Two cases of late death were reported during post-operative follow-up (3%) following heart failure within 12 months, in the first case, and at 14 months, in the second case, from an undetermined cause at home.

Post-operative echocardiography showed a decrease in the mean size of the OG compared with pre-operatively, to 31.1 cm^2 [15 - 56]. We found that 14 patients (25%) had LV dilatation, eight of whom were dysfunctional (14%). Study of the DO showed dilatation in 41 patients (74%), with a significant increase in size compared with preoperative to 18.4 cm2 ± 6.7 cm2 [9 - 41] ($p < 0.001$).

A study of the evolution of the TIA postoperatively showed that 15 patients had worsened their TIA (27%). Of these, 10 had moderate to severe IT (18%), while five others had severe IT (9%).

We also noted a significant worsening of the diameter of the tricuspid annulus postoperatively ($p<0.001$), with 35 patients having a TA> 35 mm (64%). Only one patient developed tricuspid narrowing, with moderate IT and a dilated annulus.

Among the patients who had worsened their IT after left valve surgery, five required late repeat surgery to repair tricuspid damage (9%), whether or not associated with a procedure on the left ventricle.

The remaining 10 patients with moderate to severe tricuspid insufficiency after left valve surgery (18%), in whom an indication for isolated tricuspid surgery was not established due to the presence of major PAH and/or a failing LV, were put on optimal medical treatment.

The following factors were associated with worsening TIA postoperatively: long-term anticoagulant therapy ($p = 0.008$ and OR = 18.986), the presence of more than two risk factors ($p = 0.013$ and OR = 9.457), preoperative AF ($p = 0.004$ and OR = 11.496) and preoperative LV size > 33 cm^2 ($p = 0.049$ and OR = 3.744).

2 .STRENGTHS AND LIMITATIONS OF OUR STUDY :

Our work was based on the ongoing concern about the evolution of unrepaired minimal to moderate tricuspid insufficiency after left heart valve replacements and the study of the factors influencing the worsening of this tricuspid leak over the long term.

Our series is the largest Tunisian series in terms of number of patients, investigating the factors associated with worsening of tricuspid leakage after left-sided valve surgery. Previous studies have focused mainly on mitral valve surgery, but in the present study we included patients operated on the aortic valve in order to assess the worsening of TI.

In addition, the large number of statistical tests used and the existence of identical clinical and ultrasound parameters assessed before and after the operation enabled us assess the degree of change in these parameters postoperatively.

Nevertheless, our study has a number of limitations, which are not negligible. The main limitation was the retrospective and monocentric nature of the study. The sample of patients was relatively small compared with worldwide series, which is one of the limitations that inevitably leads to a lack of power. Indeed, the relative risk of each of the associated factors was statistically unreliable given the small size of the population, apart from the frequency of worsening observed postoperatively. A prospective study with a larger number of patients would help determine the factors predictive of postoperative IT.

The fact that preoperative echocardiography was carried out by several cardiologists from different cardiology departments could bias the results, given that this is an operator-dependent test.

On the other hand, the duration of the follow-up, which is relatively short compared with worldwide series, influenced the study of the long-term evolution of IT.

3 . KEY STRENGTHS AND LIMITATIONS OF THE MAIN RESULTS IN THE LITERATURE :

The retrospective nature of most of the studies had a negative impact on the final pooled results.

Although valve surgery habits were common in the different study centres, many operators were involved during the period of the different series, and this constituted a major limitation. Indeed, the choice of surgical procedure depended on the surgeon, and some were slightly more inclined to opt for valve replacement with preservation of the sub-valvular apparatus. This conservative technique has been shown to be a protective factor against the development of postoperative IT. For this reason, in some studies, the surgeon variable has been included in the propensity score (PS) model.

In other studies, certain echographic parameters, notably LV function and annulus size, were not assessed. Further, more in-depth studies are still needed, to revise the relationship between worsening TIA and LV dysfunction or annulus dilatation.

4 .THEORETICAL BACKGROUND :

The tricuspid valve, often associated with regurgitation and once relegated to the status of "forgotten valve", is now emerging as the new focus interest. This transformation stems from its growing importance in terms of prevalence and potential severity, and from promising advances in percutaneous curative treatment techniques.

Tricuspid insufficiency was observed in approximately 80% of cardiac ultrasounds performed [18]. In the United States, 1.6 million patients had moderate to severe TIA. However, only 8,000 patients were candidates for tricuspid valve surgery [18,19].

4.1. Mechanism of tricuspid insufficiency functional :

Functional tricuspid insufficiency is characterised by ventriculoatrial regurgitation. An understanding of the pathological process of functional IT is necessary to determine the optimal management strategy for this condition.

The TA is a component of both the tricuspid valve and the VD. Dilatation of the TA occurs at the expense of its anterior and posterior parts, corresponding to the free wall of the VD (Figure 18).

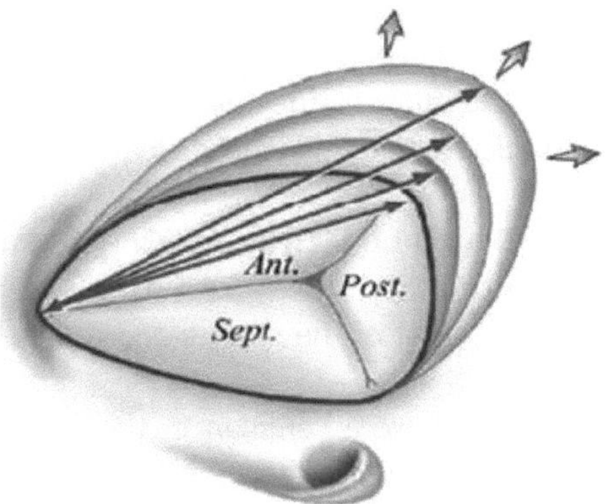

Figure 18: Pathological process of tricuspid annular dilatation [20].

Functional IT is due to valve leaflet fixation, resulting in a decrease in leaflet coaptation caused by :

Annular dilatation: This plays a predominant role in the onset of TI, following right atrial dilatation caused by AF. This is secondary to the rise in pressure in the pulmonary circulation.

Systolic kinetics of the annulus: Systolic shortening of the annulus is reduced by half in the most severe forms [21,22]. After correction of left heart valve disease, the absence of improvement in the systolic shortening of the annulus is associated with the persistence of a tachycardia.

Misalignment of the valves in systole: the maintenance of the valves in the anterior position of the annulus by the traction of the cords due to ventricular dilatation can lead to asymmetric traction.

In AF, the loss of atrial systole also contributes to regurgitation.

4.2. Consequences of functional tricuspid insufficiency :

IT increases the preload of the VD, which in most cases is already subject to increased afterload due to pulmonary hyperpressure. It thus contributes to ventricular dilatation. The pressure in the DO rises as a result of the increase in ventricular filling pressure and, above all, systolic regurgitation. This increase in pressure causes the DO to dilate.

In diastole, the pressure remains high due to impaired compliance of the VD. Atrial hyperpressure is transmitted upstream to the systemic venous circulation, resulting in an increase in venous pressures, which can lead to right heart failure. In this way, severe and long-standing IT can lead to heart failure as a result of LV dysfunction and AF.

In addition, progressive dilatation of the VD is responsible dilatation of the TA, which will increase the tachycardia. This is not always reversible after correction of the tachycardia or its cause [23,24].

4.3. Tricuspid valve surgery for tricuspid insufficiency :

As the recommendations for concomitant tricuspid valve surgery at the time of left heart valve surgery are recent, it is not uncommon to see these patients with a significant TIA at a distance from left heart surgery.

According to the latest recommendations of the European Society of Cardiology and the European Cardio-Thoracic Association revised in 2021 [2] (Appendix 4), surgery is indicated for patients with severe functional IT proposed for left heart valve surgery (Class I).

It should be considered in :

Patients with minimal to moderate secondary IT with a dilated AT (> 40 mm or > 21 mm/m^2) and proposed for left valve surgery (Class IIb).

Patients with severe functional IT, with or without previous left valve surgery, who are symptomatic or have LV dilatation, in the absence of severe right or left ventricular dysfunction or significant PAH (Class IIb).

The benefits of isolated tricuspid surgery for secondary IT compared with medical treatment are not well established, given that the surgical procedure carries a non-negligible risk of peri-operative morbidity and mortality in the event of late management [25,26].

Current European recommendations suggest curative treatment of TIA by isolated tricuspid surgery in cases of severe symptomatic TIA or impairment of right ventricular size or function, in the absence of severe LV or VD dysfunction or severe PAH [2].

5 .POPULATION PROFILE :

5.1. Age :

In several studies, age was not cited as a factor associated with worsening of CHF during follow-up of patients operated on for left heart valve disease [27,28].

However, in a meta-analysis including 11 studies, Zhu et al reported that advanced age is one of the preoperative risk factors associated with worsening of TIA after isolated left heart surgery [29].

Matsuyama et al also concluded that patients who underwent mitral valve replacement surgery and who worsened their IT postoperatively older patients [30].

In our study, the average age of the patients operated on was 50.2 ± 13.9 years, with extremes ranging from 17 to 82 years. Although the age ranges in our study were close to those reported in the literature, we did not find a significant association between advanced age and TIA (p = 0.271).

The table below illustrates the age ranges in different series in the literature.

Table XXXI: Average age according to the different series in the literature

Authors	Average age in years	Extremes (min-max)	Workforce
Song & al [4]	52	19 - 67	638
Hyung-Kwan & al [31]	45.5	17 - 69	170
Kwak & al [5]	45.2	16 - 81	335
Wang & al [32]	45.7	12 - 73	248
Our series	50.2	17 - 82	57

5.2. Genre :

Several series have highlighted the gender difference in the prediction of the course of CHF. The study by Porter et al, including 65 patients, 39 of whom (60%) were women, with rheumatic valve disease, reported an incidence of late post-operative tricuspid leakage of 67% [33]. The study was conducted on patients with significant TTI after MVR surgery and concluded that female gender was an independent factor in the worsening of TTI after left-sided valve surgery (hazard ratio 2 and RR 1.8). This female predominance associated with worsening of tricuspid leakage could be explained by the relatively high prevalence of rheumatic disease in women [34].

A Tunisian study by Bezdah et al, carried out at the Charles Nicolle Hospital, found that the incidence of severe postoperative IT was more significant in female patients (83% vs 48%; p = 0.03) [35].

This result was confirmed in a study by Gursoy et al [27]. Out of 66 patients who had undergone mitral valve surgery, 40 of whom were female (60.6%), 34 patients worsened their tricuspid leak postoperatively (51.5%) and 74.3%

of the patients were female. The analytical study concluded that female gender was an independent predictive factor for worsening of IT (p = 0.02).
In our series, there was a clear predominance of females, with a M/F sex ratio of 0.59, with no significant association with progression of IT postoperatively (p = 0.36).

5.3. Cardiovascular risk factors :

The metabolic syndrome is characterised by a series of dysfunctionsincluding insulin resistance, arterial hypertension, dyslipidaemia and obesity. In their study, Huang et al showed that this syndrome promotes degenerative valve sclerosis, which affects the tricuspid valve [32]. Mathieu et al demonstrated that these cardiovascular risk factors, being closely linked to the metabolic syndrome, are implicated in the insidious progression of valvular pathology, including the tricuspid valve [33]. Indeed, these patients showed a more rapid progression of their valvular disease because of the pro-inflammatory effects directly activated and maintained by this syndrome within the valve [34].
However, other studies have not confirmed the link between diabetes and hypertension and worsening of IT after left-sided valve surgery [28,35]. These results are consistent with our study. Indeed, the presence of more than two cardiovascular risk factors was statistically associated with a worsening of post-operative TIA (p = 0.013; OR = 9.457).

5.4. Associated pathologies:

5.4.1. Chronic renal failure (CRF) :

According to the recommendations of the French National Authority for Health (HAS), CKD is defined as creatinine clearance of less than 60 ml/min/1.73m [36].
Marwick et al have shown that the prevalence of valve disease, particularly tricuspid disease, is increased in patients CKD compared with the general population [37,38]. Garcia Fuster et al, in a study of factors in the development of late MI after mitral valve replacement, found that CKD was a predictive factor for in-hospital mortality and late mortality [40].
Despite the aforementioned results, CKD has not been shown in the literature to be a predictive factor in the development of TIA after mitral valve surgery [26,40].
In our series, only one patient had preoperative CKD (2%) which was not implicated in the progression of tricuspid leak after left valve surgery.

5.4.2. Rheumatic fever (RF):

Rheumatic disease has been described the main cause of acquired valve disease. It remains frequent in developing countries, despite prevention efforts [41]. A study by Buleu et al showed that AAR was a risk factor for the development of valvular heart disease, requiring strict long-term monitoring of

these patients [42].
In our series, 39 patients had a history of AAR from an early age.

5.5. Long-term anticoagulant treatment :

In our series, 34 patients were on long-term treatment (60%), including 28 on anticoagulants (49%) and six on antiplatelet agents (10%).
The analytical study concluded that this factor was associated with a worsening of TIA postoperatively (p = 0.008). This may be explained by the use of anticoagulants in patients with AF, which is itself associated with worsening of tricuspid leakage after left valve surgery.

5.6. Euroscore II :

Peri-operative mortality, prior to any open heart surgery, is estimated by the Euroscore II, based on well-defined clinical and ultrasound parameters of the patient [10]. A higher score predicts a greater risk of mortality.
According to the literature, the average Euroscore II varies between 0.8 and 15 for subjects proposed for valve replacement.
For patients proposed for tricuspid surgery, mean Euroscore II was 6.4% [3.8 - 10.1%], according to the study by Groger et al involving 180 patients with severe IT.
In our series, the mean Euroscore II was 2.46% [0.76% - 18.4%].

6 .ETIOLOGIES OF VALVULOPATHY :

6.1. Rheumatic :

AAR remains a frequent public health problem in developing countries, in contrast to Western countries, where it has become rare. Patients tend to be operated on at an advanced stage, due to difficulties in accessing care. This underlines the importance of prevention in improving the management of this condition [41].
According to Song et al, in a study of 638 patients in Seoul, rheumatic origin was the main cause of valvulopathy [4]. The same study concluded that rheumatic aetiology was an independent factor associated with worsening TIA after isolated left heart surgery. Similarly, Wang et al, Gursoy et al and Essayagh et al confirmed these results [25,26,40].
The mechanism by which IT worsens is thought to be related to the increased sensitivity of the left ventricle and tricuspid valve to sub-clinical damage caused by left heart valve lesions [7]. This leads to progressive right ventricular dysfunction.
In our series, although rheumatic cause was the predominant aetiology (75%), it was not shown to be a factor associated with the progression of postoperative IT.

6.2. Degenerative diseases:

Now the most common cause of acquired valve disease in Western countries, degenerative disease is often seen in the elderly. This is due to improved health conditions and increased life expectancy [39]. Degenerative damage to left heart valves often leads to functional IT due to dilatation of the TA and the VD, but also due to anchoring of the tricuspid leaflets. This structural alteration is a factor in the progression of tricuspid leakage after left heart surgery [40,41].

A study by Essayagh et al showed that degenerative mitral disease is the cause of severe functional TIA after valve surgery [42]. This was confirmed by Navia et al, in a study analysing the impact of degenerative left heart valve disease on the development of CHF [43].

In our series, degenerative disease was the second most common valvular etiology, affecting 6 patients (12%), two of whom developed moderate to severe IT during follow-up.

6.3. Other pathologies :

Infectious aetiology, aortic bicuspidism and Barlow's disease have not been reported in the literature as factors associated with worsening of tricuspid leakage after left-sided valve surgery [44].

7 .CLINICAL STUDY :

7.1. Functional signs :

7.1.1. Dyspnoea :

Dyspnoea is the main symptom of valvular patients. Its clinical presentation varies, depending on the underlying cause, ranging from progressively progressive dyspnoea to acute dyspnoea [45].

According to Gabella et al and Garcia Fuster et al, NYHA stages III and IV were predominant and were identified as a factor in hospital mortality after mitral surgery [46,47]. This is due to the fact that left heart surgery was performed at a stage of severe pulmonary hyperpressure. Because of this perioperative mortality, the prevalence of postoperative IT has been underestimated [29].

The results of our series are in line with those reported in the literature. Dyspnoea was the most frequent functional sign in our study (95%). Most patients consulted at a late stage, with 34 in stage III (60%) and 12 in stage IV (21%).

Moderate to severe IT was observed in 15 of the dyspnoeic patients postoperatively, with no significant association ($p = 0.554$).

7.1.2. Other functional signs :

Palpitations were second only to dyspnoea in frequency. They were present in 15 patients (26%) and reflected cardiac arrhythmia, underlying valvular disease or heart failure [48].

Syncope and lipothymia, on the other hand, reflect a sudden drop in cerebral output, often linked to aortic stenosis [49]. In our series, 13 patients (23%) presented with lipothymia.

The presence of these functional signs was not identified as a factor associated with worsening of tricuspid leakage after repair of left heart valve disease.

7.2. Physical signs :

7.2.1. Auscultatory abnormality :

It may be discovered incidentally during a clinical examination or during follow-up of a patient with AAR, and enables early diagnosis of valve disease before symptoms appear.

7.2.2. Signs of heart failure :

Delayed management of left-sided heart valve disease inevitably leads to left-sided heart failure in the initial phase, followed by right-sided stasis and consequent right-sided heart failure [50].

Signs of left or right heart failure reflect the severity of mitral and/or aortic valve disease and their impact on the right heart [51].

In our series, 10% of our patients were in left heart failure, reflecting the advanced stage of their valvular disease, two of whom developed moderate to severe IT after left valve surgery (p=0.606).

7.2.3. Embolic accidents :

Neurological manifestations may be the clinical presentation of valve disease. They mainly occur during an embolic event, such as a stroke or transient ischemic attack (TIA). These neurological events have usually been observed in patients with mitral stenosis [51].

In our series, two patients had preoperative hemiplegia related to ischemic stroke of embolic origin (4%).

7.3. Additional tests:

7.3.1. Chest X-ray :

Performed systematically on all patients proposed for valve surgery, this examination can reveal a number of abnormalities and raise suspicions of valve disease in patients with no known valve disease.

It may be normal or show :

- Signs of heart failure, in particular hilar overload.
- Cardiomegaly due to dilatation of the heart chambers.
- A mitral silhouette associated with progressive dilatation of the OG, OD and pulmonary artery.
- Dilation of the ascending aorta.
- Protrusion of the aortic button with calcifications.

In our series, 40 patients had cardiomegaly (70%) and 10 had hilar overload (18%), while mitral silhouette was present in 28 patients (49%).

7.3.2. Electrocardiogram :

It is used identify the various electrical abnormalities, in particular rhythm disorders, conductive disorders, ischaemic signs and signs of ventricular and atrial hypertrophy. Preoperative AF is the most studied predictive factor in published studies, given its significant involvement in the progression of IT after left-sided valve surgery [4,27,30,52]. The mechanism of worsening of postoperative CHF in patients with AF is uncertain. It has been reported that atrial dilatation leads to the onset of AF [68,69], which in turn induces persistent mechanical and electrical remodelling of both atria, leading to further atrial dilatation [53,54].

Several studies have identified preoperative AF as a determinant of the progression of CHF. It has been shown that surgical ablation concomitant with left valve surgery, in cases of recent AF, has a beneficial effect in preventing late-onset CHF [31,55].

The results of our series are in line with the literature, which concludes that AF is a factor associated with worsening of tricuspid leakage after left-sided valve surgery ($p = 0.001$).

7.3.3. Doppler ultrasound :

7.3.3.1. Trans-thoracic echocardiography (TTE) :

In patients with valvular heart disease, TTE is the gold standard. It is used to study the various parameters of the left and right heart chambers in order to make the diagnosis and assess the severity of the valve disease.

In the literature, certain echographic elements have been identified as factors associated with the progression of TIA after correction of left-sided valve disease. In decreasing order of incrimination, these factors were :

OG size :

Several publications have highlighted the fact that an increased OG surface area has been incriminated as a predictive factor for worsening tricuspid leakage after left valve surgery.

Bouchahda et al demonstrated, in a study carried out in Tunisia in patients with mitral stenosis, that a dilated OG with a lower strain was associated with more severe symptoms and tighter stenosis [56].

Matsuyama et al reported that a significantly dilated OG, following long-term LV volume or pressure overload, probably associated with AF, may contribute to the development of IT [30].

Data from the Framingham and Strong Heart population studies showed that a dilated OG was an independent predictor of AF, leading to progression of tricuspid leak after left valve surgery [57,58].

Our results are consistent with those reported in the literature. All patients who worsened their TTI postoperatively had a dilated LV (>20 cm^2) (Figure

19). In our series, an OG size > 33 cm2 was identified as an independent factor associated with worsening of tricuspid leakage postoperatively (p = 0.049; OR = 3.744).

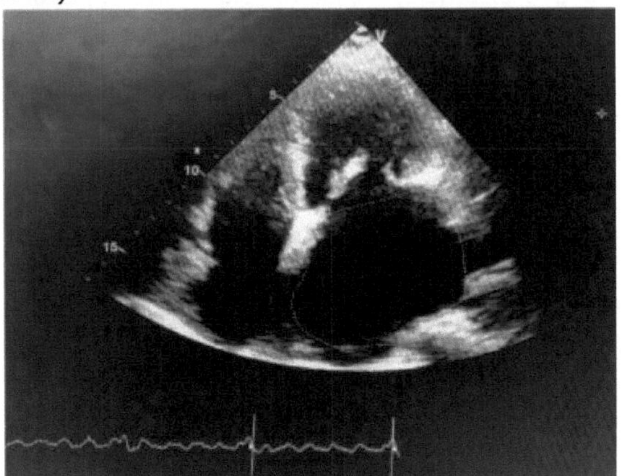

Figure 19: Ultrasound image of a dilated left atrium

OD size :

Wang et al found that a dilated DO can worsen tricuspid leak after left-sided valve surgery [32]. This was confirmed by the study of Vaturi et al, who deduced that increased DO surface area was responsible for dilatation of the TA, and consequently progression of TI over time [59].

This hypothesis was invalidated by a meta-analysis by Zhu et al, who proposed that the size of the DO should be studied by more parameters and did not identify it as a predictive factor for worsening TIA [29].

In our series, the size of the DO was not identified as a factor associated with the progression of IT postoperatively (p = 0.061).

Moderate preoperative IT :

Repair of a significant TIA is the rule, but correction of a minimal to moderate TIA remains controversial.

Previously, if the TA was not judged to be dilated during surgery, even in the presence of a moderate TIA, plastic surgery was not indicated. This was justified by the idea of a reduction in VD overload, and therefore a spontaneous regression of TIA after left heart surgery.

Recent studies have ruled out this theory. Matsuyama et al showed that moderate IT worsened in 37% of patients after left valve surgery. The authors of this study suggested that this progression was associated with preoperative LV dysfunction [30].

Navia et al analysed 1,724 subjects operated on for left-sided degenerative valve disease with a moderate TIA, divided into two groups with or without

TIA repair. 15% of patients with unrepaired moderate valve disease developed significant postoperative valve disease in the second group, compared with 7% in the first group (p<0.0001), over a 3-year follow-up period [43].
Bezdah et al conducted a study of 56 patients who had undergone left heart surgery with or without tricuspid annuloplasty. This study found that 23% of patients developed significant TIA postoperatively. The presence of minimal to moderate preoperative TI was a predictor of worsening of postoperative tricuspid leak (p = 0.04) [35].
In their meta-analysis, Zhu et al confirmed the role of moderate IT in the development of postoperative tricuspid leak, with an OR almost twice as high [29].
The results of our series found that the presence of minimal to moderate IT (Figure 20) preoperatively was not significantly associated with IT progression (p = 0.749).

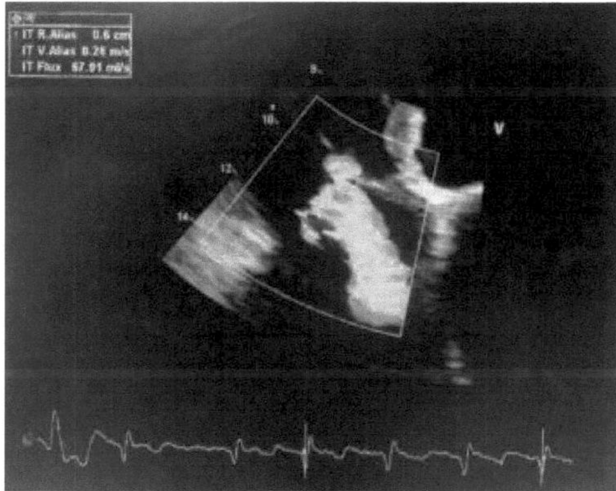

Figure 20: Ultrasound image of moderate tricuspid insufficiency

Tricuspid ring :
According to the literature, the diameter of the annulus has been found to associated with the development of significant late IT. Indeed, once the TA is dilated, its size continues to evolve further. This condition explains the tendency for TIA to worsen in some patients after right heart surgery [20,60].
Porter et al demonstrated that the dilatation of the TA was more reliable than the degree of TIA when studying the progression of functional TIA. They considered that the diameter of the TA was important in the decision to repair minimal to moderate TIAs [33,60].
Song et al demonstrated that the TA significantly increased in size in patients who developed significant TIA after left-sided valve surgery [4]. However, this study failed to identify the predictive value of preoperative TA size in the progression of TIA.

Another study by Takano et al studying the incrimination of TA in the indication for tricuspid plasty during left valve surgery concluded that the size of the tricuspid annulus preoperatively was not a valid parameter, as commonly agreed [61].

A recent report by Colombo et al indicated that TA dilatation with systolic annular size reduction, reflecting LV dysfunction, is associated with a poor prognosis [62].

Our analytical study did not find TA size to be a factor associated with this worsening ($p = 0.171$).

VG function :

Preoperative ejection fraction has not been shown to be a factor in the worsening of significant postoperative TIA. However, the majority of these studies involved patients with normal or slightly decreased ejection fraction [5,32,34,63]. Further studies are therefore needed to evaluate patients with moderate or severe left ventricular dysfunction [27].

In our series, LV function was impaired in only nine patients (16%) and was not significantly associated with the development of tricuspid leakage ($p = 0.692$).

Mitral surface :

A prospective Tunisian study carried out at the military hospital by Taamallah et al found that the tighter the mitral surface, the more impaired the function of the VD ($p < 0.05$) [64].

In our study, we found that mitral surface area $< 1cm^2$ was statistically associated with worsening of postoperative IT with $p = 0.032$.

Function and size of the VD :

The size and function of the VD are closely linked to the development of TI [65,66]. The question was whether preoperative LV dysfunction or dilatation predicts the development of late TIA after left-sided valve surgery.

Zhu et al took these parameters into consideration, but due to the paucity of studies in the literature including these ultrasound data, preoperative right ventricular dilatation and dysfunction were not included in the worsening of IT [29].

In addition, patients with minimal to moderate TIA had preserved preoperative LV size and function. These were not considered to be significant predictors of late TIA [67].

In our series, LV function and size were not significantly associated with worsening of IT postoperatively ($p = 0.714$; $p = 0.298$ respectively).

PAH :

Studies by Matsuyama and Porter have shown that in some patients, preoperative PAH due to mitral valve disease does not always tend to regress after left heart surgery. Persistent pulmonary overload may lead to progression of IT [30,33].

Wang et al found, in their study of 248 patients, that 37.3% of patients with preoperative PAH developed a significant IT [32]. This criterion was not a factor associated with worsening of tricuspid leak.

The study by Song et al confirms these results [4].

In our series, 51 patients had preoperative PAH, 10 of whom had major PAH (18%). Only one of these patients developed significant IT after left valve repair surgery. Statistical analysis did not find PAH to be a factor associated with worsening TIA (p=1).

7.3.3.2. Trans-oesophageal echocardiography (TEE:

TEE is an essential adjunct to TTE in many situations involving valvular pathology that is poorly explored by TTE. The main indications include endocarditis, detection of intra-atrial thrombi, intraoperative considerations and assessment of the severity of valve damage, in particular the mechanism of mitral insufficiency, or prosthetic , in particular exploration of stenosis or thrombosis or a paraprosthetic leak [68].

8 .SURGICAL TREATMENT :

8.1. Extracorporeal circulation :

A study by Denault et al showed that a longer duration of CEC in valve replacements could lead to dysfunction and dilation of the VD and subsequently dilation of the tricuspid annulus [69].

Conversely, Song et al did not find the duration of bypass surgery or aortic clamping to be predictive factors for worsening TIA after left valve surgery [4].

In our series, the mean duration of CEC and aortic clamping were not significantly associated with the worsening of IT postoperatively.

8.2. Valvular gesture :

8.2.1. Mitral valve :

A number of studies have found that isolated mitral valve replacement in patients minimal to moderate CHF is predictive of worsening CHF postoperatively and may even lead to repeat surgery [33,52,61].

Mitral plasty :

Although conservative techniques have evolved, mitral plasty was not always feasible [70] due to remodelling and calcification of the leaflets and cords or in the presence of extensive lesions of infective endocarditis [17].

A study by Matsunga et al, involving 70 patients with ischaemic mitral insufficiency associated with minimal to moderate IT, found worsening of IT in more than half after conservative mitral surgery [52].

In our study, only one patient out of the three who had undergone mitral plasty required a repeat operation because the plasty had become stenotic and the tricuspid leak had worsened (p = 1).

Mitral valve replacement :

In cases of rheumatic disease with significant valvular and subvalvular changes, conservative surgery is not possible. Mitral valve replacement is performed with the aim of preserving the sub-valvular apparatus, given its value in preserving left ventricular function [71].

In our series, 13 patients who had undergone mitral valve replacement worsened their IT postoperatively. The latter was not significantly associated with this worsening (p = 0.304).

8.2.2. Aortic valve :

Aortic valve replacement is the gold standard treatment for patients with symptomatic aortic disease. It is a simple procedure, often without complications. However, careful intraoperative handling of calcifications is essential avoid any incidents.

Wang et al demonstrated, in their study analysing the factors predictive of IT secondary to left valve surgery, that aortic valve replacement was associated with a significant worsening of tricuspid leakage postoperatively (p = 0.001). This was noted in four out of 41 patients [32].

In our study, six of the 25 patients who underwent aortic valve replacement worsened their IT postoperatively, without being significantly associated with this progression (p = 0.739).

8.2.3. Multiple valve procedures :

Polyvalvulopathy can occur in a number of conditions, in particular rheumatic diseases, but also degenerative diseases.

In the literature, there is no clear consensus regarding the surgical management of multiple valve lesions [72,73]. In fact, the surgical decision may prove difficult when faced with double mitro-aortic valve disease, one of which was initially assessed as moderate to moderate and which may subsequently have an impact on the right heart if it has not been repaired [2].

A study by Wang et al found that the incidence of secondary TIA after left-sided valve surgery was greater with multiple than isolated valve procedures [32].

In our series, of the 13 patients who underwent double mitro-aortic replacement, eight developed moderate to severe IT postoperatively, without being significantly associated with worsening of the tricuspid leak (p = 0.31).

9 .CARE IN INTENSIVE CARE UNITS :

9.1. Postoperative morbidity :

9.1.1. Rhythm disorders :

Kalra et al found a 50% incidence of postoperative onset AF after aortic or mitral valve surgery, with significantly higher in-hospital mortality in these patients [74].

Kim et al studied the importance of surgical ablation of AF, associated with left valve surgery, in preventing the complications of arrhythmias, namely heart failure, embolic accidents [75], maintenance of sinus rhythm, but also the progression of IT postoperatively [55].

In our series, atrial fibrillation was the most frequent postoperative complication observed in 31 patients (54%). Univariate analysis found postoperative AF to be a factor significantly associated with worsening tricuspid leakage after left-sided valve surgery (p = 0.002).

9.1.2. Postoperative infectious pneumonitis :

In the literature, infectious pneumonitis has been described as a frequent complication after valve surgery, with an incidence varying between 2.8 and 23% [76,77].

This condition was found to be strongly associated with high postoperative mortality. The various factors predictive of postoperative pneumonitis cited in several studies were the presence of metabolic syndrome, impaired LV ejection fraction, chronic renal failure and surgery in an emergency setting [78,79].

In our series, more than half the patients (51%) developed postoperative pneumonitis, a relatively high incidence compared with that described in the literature, although it was not associated with postoperative progression of IT (p = 0.956).

9.1.3. Bleeding complications :

Postoperative bleeding is a concern for all patients undergoing extracorporeal circulation, with an incidence of up to 12% [80].

Bleeding after surgery may be due to surgical causes or to a biological imbalance following bypass surgery, with consumption of coagulation factors, altered platelet function and activation of fibrinolysis [81].

Biological bleeding :

Hall et al found that postoperative coagulopathy complicated by bleeding was more frequent in patients treated preoperatively with heparin (37%; p = 0.052). They also showed that prolonged clamping and bypass times and redux surgery were predictive factors of postoperative biological bleeding (p =0.001) [80].

In this context, bleeding is often controlled by the administration of blood products and derivatives.

In our population, bleeding related to haemostasis disorders was not incriminated in the progression of postoperative IT (p=1).

Surgical bleeding :

Tamponade is a complication associated with increased perioperative morbidity and mortality [82,83].

In the event of surgical bleeding, it is important to determine the indication and the time frame for resumption. Kirklin and Barrat-Boyes have proposed protocols to be followed when deciding whether to repeat surgery, based on the amount of blood drained and the kinetics of the bleeding [81,82].

In our series, three patients (5%) were reoperated for postoperative bleeding. This was not associated with the occurrence of late IT (p=1).

9.1.4. Conductive disorders :

Conduction disorders are one of the most serious complications following valve surgery, caused by lesions in the conduction pathways. Depending on the study, this risk varies from 7 to 15% [86].

Several studies have identified age, AF, prosthesis size and mitral valve surgery as risk factors in the occurrence of postoperative AVB [87,88].

The latter may be transient or permanent. There are no criteria for predicting reversibility [89].

In our series, the occurrence of postoperative conduction disorders was not associated with a worsening of the IT postoperatively (p=0.071).

9.1.5. Parietal infections :

Mediastinitis is a potentially fatal complication after median sternotomy, with an incidence of 1 to 5% [90]. Patients with deep parietal infection had twice mortality rate of patients without mediastinitis, with in-hospital mortality ranging from 10 to 47% [91].

Parietal infections, known as superficial infections, require regular local care with or without antibiotic therapy, depending on the severity of the infection. Nevertheless, they must be diagnosed and treated in good time to avoid developing into mediastinitis [90,92].

In our series, of the three patients who developed a parietal infection, only one patient had a worsening of his postoperative IT, with no statistically significant association (2%; p = 1).

9.2. Postoperative mortality :

Garcia Fuster et al found in their study a peri-operative mortality rate for left heart surgery of 5.5%. The main causes of postoperative death were cardiogenic shock, infectious pneumonitis, multivisceral failure and infective endocarditis [47].

No cases of immediate post-operative hospital death were reported in our study.

10 . POST-OPERATIVE FOLLOW-UP :

10.1. Reverse :

In our study, the mean follow-up time between surgery and the last consultation was 42.1 months, with extremes ranging from 12 to 67 months.

The follow-up period was shorter than in the literature, given the delayed emergence of cardiac surgery in our country and the smaller number of patients.

The table below compares the postoperative follow-up with that reported in the literature.

Table XXXII: Length of literature compared to that in the setback

Study	Country	n	Time to recoil (months)
Garcia Fuster **[47]**	Spain	801	85.2 [16 - 192]
Di Mauro **[93]**	Italy	165	28 [11 - 60]
Chan **[94]**	Canada	450	81.6 ± 57.6
Ariyochi **[28]**	Japan	52	55.2 ± 32.4
Our series	Tunisia	57	42.1 [12 - 72]

10.2. Remote mortality :

A study by Takano et al on the occurrence of late IT after mitral surgery found a mortality rate of 16.03% following sepsis, heart failure, pneumonia or cerebral haemorrhage [61].

Another study by Kwak et al, looking at the development of significant tricuspid leakage after left-sided valve surgery, found 62 late postoperative deaths among 335 patients, giving a mortality rate of 18.5%. The leading causes of distant mortality were heart failure, stroke, myocardial infarction and endocarditis [5].

During our post-operative follow-up, two cases of late death were reported (4%). We noted a lower mortality rate than in the literature.

10.3. Clinical course :

10.3.1. Dyspnoea :

Dyspnoea has been reported to be the main symptom in patients undergoing mitral valve replacement who develop significant IT postoperatively. These results were confirmed by Li et al, with 26 patients (57.8%) in NYHA stage III and 19 others in stage IV (42.9%) [95].

In our series, post-operative follow-up showed a statistically significant total regression of dyspnoea postoperatively (p=0.013). Of the patients who continued to suffer from dyspnoea (73%), we noted an improvement in 10 patients (18%) from NHYA stage III to stage II.

10.3.2. Other symptoms :

Apart from dyspnoea, no other symptoms have been reported in the literature.

In our study, late symptoms other than dyspnoea were related to prosthesis-related complications. Three patients had late lipothymia related to aortic stenosis. We also noted a postoperative syncopal episode related to thrombosis of an aortic prosthesis.

10.4. Ultrasound evolution :

10.4.1. Assessment of postoperative tricuspid insufficiency :

Study of tricuspid leakage :

The evolution of a late IT resulted in significant postoperative morbidity and mortality despite correction of the underlying left heart valve disease [96].

The table below compares the evolution of postoperative tricuspid leak in several studies.

Table XXXIII: Comparison of the evolution of postoperative tricuspid leak with that in the literature

Study	Country	n	Worsening of IT	Severe IT
Izumi et al [96]	**Japan**	**208**	14%	3.7%
Kwak et al [5]	**South Korea**	**335**	26.9%	7.5%
Song et al [4]	**South Korea**	**584**	6.26%	1.41%
Bezdah et al [35]	**Tunisia**	**56**	23%	-
Our series	**Tunisia**	**57**	27%	9%

Our results are similar to those reported in the literature. The study of the tricuspid valve after left-sided valve surgery showed that 15 patients worsened their initially minimal to moderate IT after left-sided valve surgery (27%). Of these patients, ten became moderate to severe (18%), and a further five had severe TIA (9%).

Study of the tricuspid annulus :

Takano et al compared the size of the TA before and after left-sided valve surgery in two groups of patients with minimal to moderate IT who were not operated on by the same surgeon. The first group underwent tricuspidoplasty, while the second did not [61]. This study found that patients who did not have a tricuspid procedure increased the size of the indexed TA during the follow-up period, whereas in the others, the size of the TA decreased.

In our series, we noted a significant worsening of the diameter of the tricuspid annulus postoperatively, i.e. $p < 0.001$, of which 35 patients were found to have a TA> 35 mm (64%) compared with eight preoperatively.

None of the patients with an AT > 35mm and < 40 mm preoperatively worsened their TIA postoperatively, whereas 15 of the patients with an AT < 35 mm preoperatively worsened their TIA (Figure 21).

All preoperative patients had an indexed TA< 21 mm/m^2. Postoperatively, 15 patients had an indexed TA > 21 mm/m^2 (27%).

The size of the band was not a factor significantly associated with worsening of postoperative IT (p = 0.171).

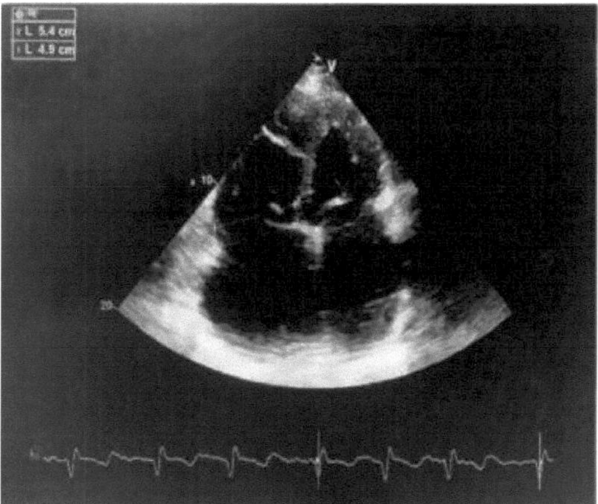

Figure 21: Ultrasound image of a dilated tricuspid annulus

10.4.2. Study of the haemodynamic profile of prostheses :

Paraprosthetic leaks can occur before the annulus has completely healed. However, disinsertion of the prosthesis may complicate surgery, following endocarditis or suture on fragile tissue [97,98].

The major risk of implantation of mechanical prostheses is thrombosis. This occurs mainly as a result of unadjusted doses of VKA or poor compliance with anticoagulant treatment by the patient [99].

A study of the haemodynamic profile of the prostheses in our series found that the number of stenosing prostheses in the mitral position was five (9%) (Figure 22) and two in the aortic position (4%). In contrast, mitral and aortic paraprosthetic leaks were noted in three patients (5%) and four (7%) respectively. Only one case of thrombosis of mitral and aortic mechanical prostheses was described as a result of poor compliance with VKA.

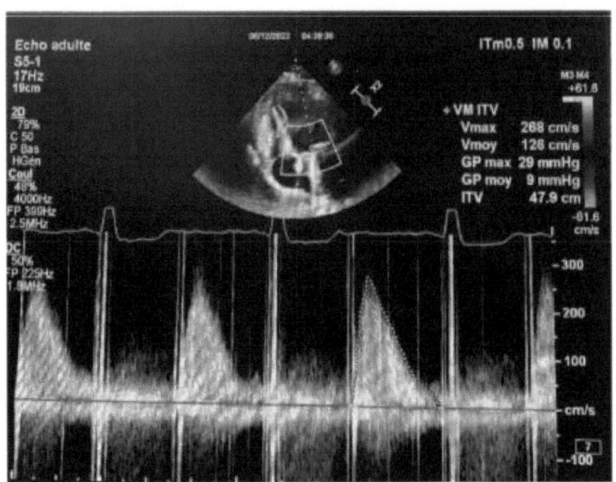

Figure 22: Ultrasound image of a stenotic mechanical mitral prosthesis

10.5. Management of patients developing moderate to severe IT with high procedural risk :

The choice of treatment for a TTI depends on its aetiology and severity. Medical treatment has been initiated for tricuspid leaks secondary to left-sided valve disease. It is based on adequate control of fluid overload and symptoms of heart failure. It is also important to educate patients to reduce their salt intake.

Digitalis, diuretics, converting enzyme inhibitors and anticoagulants are the usual treatment prescribed for these patients. Anti-arrhythmics are added as required to control AF [100].

In our series, 10 of the 15 patients with moderate to severe tricuspid insufficiency were put on medical treatment because of the presence of congestive heart failure or significant PAH.

10.6. Management of patients developing severe IT with low procedural risk :

Re-operation may be necessary in patients who have had initial left heart surgery complicated by severe IT, with a low procedural risk.

A study by Zairi et al was carried out at the Habib Thameur Hospital in Tunisia, and involved patients who had initially undergone surgery on the mitral and/or aortic valve with a minimal non-surgical CHF. Of these patients, 32 worsened their IT over a follow-up period of 23 years and required re-operation for correction of the tricuspid defect [101]. Analysis of the results showed that 68.75% of patients had moderate to severe leakage and 31.25% had severe leakage. This study identified female gender, dilated OG and the presence of AF as independent predictive factors for the progression of IT

after left-sided valve surgery.
Another study carried out in China between 1996 and 2008 included 45 patients operated on for mitral valve replacement who required repeat surgery for severe IT during their follow-up [95]. Eleven patients underwent tricuspid annuloplasty (24.4%) and 34 others underwent tricuspid valve replacement (75.5%).
In a study carried out at the Hedi Chaker Hospital in Sfax, Charfeddine et al compared the results of two tricuspid plasty techniques. This study found that DeVega plasty was a predictive factor for recurrent TIA after tricuspid repair surgery (OR = 3.26). Carpentier annuloplasty, on the other hand, seems to guarantee better postoperative results [102].
Although the procedural risk was low, peri-operative mortality remains high after redux surgery. Jeganathan et al found that late reoperation for severe IT in patients with right heart failure was associated with significant perioperative mortality [103,104].
In our series, five patients required repeat surgery to repair tricuspid damage (9%), with or without a procedure on the left heart. These patients had severe IT not associated with severe VD dysfunction or significant PAH.
Of these five patients, four underwent tricuspid annuloplasty associated with a left-sided valve procedure, either following dysfunction of the mitro-aortic prostheses in one patient, or mitral plasty that became stenotic in a second, or the appearance of new left-sided heart valve disease in the other two.
Only one patient had an isolated procedure on the tricuspid valve in the form of tricuspid valve replacement by bioprosthesis, resulting in a tricuspid narrowing associated with the initial insufficiency, thought to be of rheumatic origin.
All these patients undergoing re-operation had preoperative AF on long-term treatment, rheumatic valve disease and an OG > 33 cm^2 on TTE.
The following factors were associated with worsening TIA postoperatively: long-term anticoagulant therapy ($p = 0.008$ and OR = 18.986), the presence of more than two risk factors ($p = 0.013$ and OR = 9.457), preoperative AF ($p = 0.004$ and OR = 11.496) and preoperative LV size > 33 cm^2 ($p = 0.049$ and OR = 3.744).
Based on the data in the literature and the results of our study, minimal to moderate functional IT associated with unrepaired left heart valve disease may worsen and present late, making further surgery difficult.
The ESC recommendations for minimal to moderate functional TR are limited to dilatation of the TA> 40mm or > 21 mm/m2 associated with left heart valve disease. However, this unrepaired tricuspid leak may evolve on its own after left-sided valve surgery and require reintervention, the morbi-mortality of

which is not negligible.

These results have been confirmed in the literature, by studying the factors associated with this aggravation, which essentially include female gender, rheumatic aetiology, preoperative atrial fibrillation and preoperative dilated OG.

In our country, rheumatic disease is still endemic, despite modest preventive efforts. Although in our series, rheumatic aetiology was not a factor associated with postoperative worsening of TI, it should be taken into consideration in the management of minimal to moderate tricuspid leaks.

This pathology, which is a major cause of morbidity and mortality, leads to right ventricular dysfunction, which is compounded by the high frequency of postoperative pneumopathy and the significant costs involved. It is therefore appropriate to adopt a fairly aggressive approach by acting on minimal to moderate functional IT at the time of left heart surgery, in the presence of these predictive factors.

5 CONCLUSIONS

For a long time, the functional tricuspid leak concomitant with left heart valve disease was not repaired, due to the predominant theory that it improved after left heart surgery. This hypothesis has been called into question, due to the unpredictable evolution of minimal to moderate tricuspid leakage not considered surgical during correction of left heart valve disease.

The objectives of our work were to study the evolution of unrepaired minimal to moderate tricuspid insufficiency after left heart surgery and to identify factors associated with worsening of tricuspid leakage after left heart valve surgery.

We conducted a retrospective, descriptive, monocentric, longitudinal study from January 2018 to December 2022 in the cardiovascular surgery department of the Abderrahmen Mami University Hospital in Ariana.

We included 57 patients operated on for left heart valve disease associated with minimal to moderate tricuspid leakage that was not considered surgical preoperatively and postoperatively. We did not include patients who had undergone a procedure on the tricuspid valve, surgery on the ascending aorta or associated coronary surgery. We considered the clinical and echographic evolution of patients after repair of left-sided valve damage as the primary endpoint.

In our series, the average age of patients was 50.2 ± 13.9 years, with a clear predominance of women (63%).

The main cardiovascular risk factors studied in our series were arterial hypertension (17%), smoking (25%), dyslipidaemia (14%) and diabetes (12%). The majority of patients had at least two cardiovascular risk factors (37%).

A total of 34 patients were on long-term treatment (60%), including 28 on anticoagulants (49%) and six on antiplatelet agents (11%).

Rheumatic valve disease the most common aetiology. It was present in 43 patients (75%), followed by degenerative pathology in 7 patients (12%), then infective endocarditis in 5 patients (9%).

The main functional sign was dyspnoea, found in 54 of the patients in our series (95%). Stage III of the NYHA classification was predominant in 34 patients (60%), followed by stage IV in 21%.

Rhythm disorders were the most frequent electrical signs, including 29 patients with complete atrial fibrillation (51%).

A study of the ultrasound parameters found that 51 patients had OG dilatation (89%) with a mean size of 33.1 cm^2 [17 - 52]. Right ventricular dilatation was observed in five patients (9%) and LV dysfunction in three (5%). In addition, OD dilatation was observed in 30 patients (53%) with a mean size of 14.8

cm2 [10 - 29]. Severe PAH was observed in 12 patients (21%) with a mean of 50.4 mmHg [23-80].
The valvular study showed that mitral valve involvement was predominant, present in 49 patients (86%). Aortic involvement was observed in 25 cases (44%).
All patients had minimal to moderate tricuspid insufficiency preoperatively, of whom 49 had a TA < 35 mm (86%), while a further 8 had a TA> 35 mm and <40 mm (14%).
All patients were operated on under CEC with aortic clamping. Mitral valve replacement was performed in 42 patients (74%), while aortic valve replacement was performed in 25 patients (44%).
Early postoperative complications were observed in 48 patients, representing an overall morbidity of 84%.
Of the 57 patients operated on, seven experienced post-operative bleeding (12%), three of whom required repeat surgery to check haemostasis (5%).
Two patients, who were in sinus rhythm before the operation, went into AF post-operatively, and two others presented a conductive disorder of the transient 3rd degree AVB type (3%). Post-operative infectious pneumonitis was observed in 51% of patients.
The average length of stay in intensive care was 3 days [2-9]. The total length of hospital stay was 11 days [6-26].
No cases of peri-operative mortality were reported in our study.
All patients contacted for post-operative follow-up. The mean follow-up time between surgery and the last consultation was 42.1 months.
Two cases of late death were reported during post-operative follow-up (3%) following heart failure within 12 months, in the first case, and at 14 months, in the second case, from an undetermined cause at home.
Post-operative echocardiography showed a decrease in the mean size of the OG compared with pre-operatively, to 31.1 cm^2 [15 - 56]. We found that 14 patients (25%) had LV dilatation, eight of whom were dysfunctional (14%). Study of the DO showed dilatation in 41 patients (74%), with a significant increase in size compared with preoperative at 18.4 cm2 ± [9 - 41] ($p < 0.001$).
In addition, we noted a significant improvement in mean pulmonary artery pressures postoperatively compared with preoperatively with a $p<0.001$, although eight patients presented with severe PAH postoperatively (14%).
A study of the evolution of the TIA postoperatively showed that 15 patients had worsened their TIA (27%). Of these, 10 had moderate to severe IT (18%), while five others had severe IT (9%).
We also noted a significant worsening of the diameter of the tricuspid annulus

postoperatively ($p < 0.001$), with 35 patients having a TA> 35 mm (64%). Only one patient developed tricuspid narrowing, with moderate IT and a dilated annulus.
Among the patients who had worsened their IT after left valve surgery, five required late repeat surgery to repair tricuspid damage (9%), whether or not associated with a procedure on the left ventricle.
The remaining 10 patients with moderate to severe tricuspid insufficiency after left valve surgery (18%), in whom an indication for isolated tricuspid surgery was not established due to the presence of major PAH and/or a failing LV, were put on optimal medical treatment.
The following factors were associated with worsening TIA postoperatively: long-term anticoagulant therapy ($p = 0.008$ and OR = 18.986), the presence of more than two risk factors ($p = 0.013$ and OR = 9.457), preoperative AF ($p = 0.004$ and OR = 11.496) and preoperative LV size > 33 cm^2 ($p = 0.049$ and OR = 3.744).
Based on our study and the various series analysed, the evolution of unrepaired functional tricuspid insufficiency after left-sided valve surgery is associated with high short- and long-term morbidity and mortality. This is due to the need for re-intervention for severe tricuspid leakage, in several cases reported in the literature. Recent cohorts have studied the factors associated with the worsening of this IT, initially to a minimal to moderate degree, and have essentially found female gender, rheumatic aetiology, preoperative atrial fibrillation and preoperative dilated OG to be predictive factors of this unfavourable evolution.
The main limitation of our study was that it was retrospective and monocentric. In addition, the sample of patients was relatively small compared with worldwide series, which is one of the limitations that inevitably leads to a lack of power.
European recommendations have focused mainly on the indications for severe functional tricuspid insufficiency associated with left-sided valve surgery. However, in the presence of minimal to moderate CHF, the indications for tricuspid repair surgery remain controversial. Hence the need for a clear consensus, in order avoid complications linked to aggravation.

REFERENCES

1. Topilsky Y, Maltais S, Medina Inojosa J, Oguz D, Michelena H, Maalouf J, et al. Burden of tricuspid regurgitation in patients diagnosed in the community setting. JACC Cardiovasc Imaging. 2019 Mar;12(3):433-42.
2. Vahanian A, Beyersdorf F, Praz F, Milojevic M, Baldus S, Bauersachs J, et al. 2021 (ESC/EACTS) guidelines for the management of valvular heart disease. Eur Heart J. 2022 Feb;43(7):561-632.
3. Dreyfus J, Messika Zeitoun D. Tricuspid insufficiency and left valvulopathy [Online]. Cardiologie Pratique [cited 05/12/2023]; Available from URL: https://www.cardiologie- pratique.com/journal/article/0031821-insuffisance-tricuspide- valvulopathie-gauche
4. Song H, Kim MJ, Chung CH, Choo SJ, Song MG, Song JM, et al. Factors associated with development of late significant tricuspid regurgitation after successful left sided valve surgery. Heart. 2009 Jun;95(11):931-6.
5. Kwak JJ, Kim YJ, Kim MK, Kim HK, Park JS, Kim KH, et al. Development of tricuspid regurgitation late after left sided valve surgery: a single center experience with long term echocardiographic examinations. Am Heart J. 2008 Apr;155(4):732-7.
6. Braunwald NS, Ross J, Morrow AG. Conservative management of tricuspid regurgitation in patients undergoing mitral valve replacement. Circulation. 1967 Apr;35 Suppl4:S63-9.
7. Asano K, Washio M, Eguchi S. Results of mitral valve replacement, with special reference to the functional tricuspid insufficiency. Jpn Heart J. 1971 Nov;12(6):507-16.
8. Calafiore AM, Gallina S, Iacò AL, Contini M, Bivona A, Gagliardi M, et al. Mitral valve surgery for functional mitral regurgitation: should moderate or more tricuspid regurgitation be treated? a propensity score analysis. Ann Thorac Surg. 2009 Mar;87(3):698-703.
9. Iung B, Delgado V, Rosenhek R, Price S, Prendergast B, Wendler O, et al. Contemporary presentation and management of valvular heart disease the (EURObservational) research programme valvular heart disease II survey. Circulation. 2019 Oct;140(14):1156-69.
10. Nashef SAM, Roques F, Sharples LD, Nilsson J, Smith C, Goldstone AR, et al (EuroSCORE II). Eur J Cardiothorac Surg. 2012 Apr;41(4):734-45.
11. Lang RM, Badano LP, Mor Avi V, Afilalo J, Armstrong A, Ernande L, et al. Recommendations for cardiac chamber quantification by echocardiography in adults: an update from the American society of echocardiography and the European association of cardiovascular imaging. J Am Soc Echocardiogr. 2015 Jan;28(1):1-39.
12. Rudski LG, Lai WW, Afilalo J, Hua L, Handschumacher MD,

Chandrasekaran K, et al. Guidelines for the echocardiographic assessment of the right heart in adults: a report from the american society of echocardiography endorsed by the european association of echocardiography, a registered branch of the european society of cardiology, and the canadian society of echocardiography. J Am Soc Echocardiogr. 2010 Jul;23(7):685- 713.

13. Zoghbi WA, Adams D, Bonow RO, Enriquez Sarano M, Foster E, Grayburn PA, et al. Recommendations for noninvasive evaluation of native valvular regurgitation: a report from the american society of echocardiography developed in collaboration with the society for cardiovascular magnetic resonance. J Am Soc Echocardiogr. 2017 Apr;30(4):303-71.

14. Baumgartner H, Hung J, Bermejo J, Chambers JB, Evangelista A, Griffin BP, et al. Echocardiographic assessment of valve stenosis: (EAE/ASE) recommendations for clinical practice. J Am Soc Echocardiogr. 2009 Jan;22(1):1-23.

15. Jougon J, Thumerel M, Rodriguez A, Delcambre F. Anterior surgical approaches surgical approaches of the thorax and cervicothoracic. EMC - Techniques chirurgicales - Thorax 2014;31(1):1-30 [Article 42-210]

16. Clinique Saint Augustin. Sternotomy, cardiac surgery [Online]. Clinique Saint Augustin [cited 20/10/2023]; Available from the URL: https://www.chircard-iac.com/ interventions/sternotomy/

17. Chauvaud S. Surgery for acquired tricuspid valve lesions. EMC - Techniques chirurgicales - Thorax 2019;37(1):1-10 [Article 42-540]

18. Vassileva CM, Shabosky J, Boley T, Markwell S, Hazelrigg S. Tricuspid valve surgery: the past 10 years from the nationwide inpatient sample (NIS) database. J Thorac Cardiovasc Surg. 2012 May;143(5):1043-9.

19. Fender EA, Zack CJ, Nishimura RA. Isolated tricuspid regurgitation: outcomes and therapeutic interventions. Heart. 2018 May;104(10):798-806.

20. Dreyfus GD, Corbi PJ, Chan KMJ, Bahrami T. Secondary tricuspid regurgitation or dilatation: which should be the criteria for surgical repair? Ann Thorac Surg. 2005 Jan;79(1):127-32.

21. Ubago JL, Figueroa A, Ochoteco A, Colman T, Duran RM, Duran CG. Analysis of the amount of tricuspid valve anular dilatation required to produce functional tricuspid regurgitation. Am J Cardiol. 1983 Jul;52(1):155-8.

22. Tei C, Pilgrim JP, Shah PM, Ormiston JA, Wong M. The tricuspid valve annulus: study of size and motion in normal subjects and in patients with tricuspid regurgitation. Circulation. 1982 Sep;66(3):665-71.

23. Sadeghi HM, Kimura BJ, Raisinghani A, Blanchard DG, Mahmud E, Fedullo PF, et al. Does lowering pulmonary arterial pressure eliminate severe

functional tricuspid regurgitation: insights from pulmonary thromboendarterectomy. J Am Coll Cardiol. 2004 Jul;44(1):126-32.
24. Xanthopoulos A, Starling RC, Kitai T, Triposkiadis F. Heart failure and liver disease: cardiohepatic interactions. JACC Heart Fail. 2019 Feb;7(2):87-97.
25. Wang N, Fulcher J, Abeysuriya N, McGrady M, Wilcox I, Celermajer D, et al. Tricuspid regurgitation is associated with increased mortality independent of pulmonary pressures and right heart failure: a systematic review and meta analysis. Eur Heart J. 2019 Feb;40(5):476-84.
26. Zack CJ, Fender EA, Chandrashekar P, Reddy YNV, Bennett CE, Stulak JM, et al. National trends and outcomes in isolated tricuspid valve surgery. J Am Coll Cardiol. 2017 Dec;70(24):2953- 60.
27. Gursoy M, Bakuy V, Hatemi AC, Bulut G, Kilicsekmez K, Ince N, et al. Long term prognosis of mild functional tricuspid regurgitation after mitral valve replacement: an observational retrospective study. Anadolu Kardiyol Derg. 2014 Feb;14(1):34- 9.
28. Ariyoshi T, Hashizume K, Taniguchi S, Miura T, Matsukuma S, Nakaji S, et al. Which type of secondary tricuspid regurgitation accompanying mitral valve disease should be surgically treated? Ann Thorac Cardiovasc Surg. 2013 Jun;19(6):428-34.
29. Zhu TY, Min XP, Zhang HB, Meng X. Preoperative risk factors for residual tricuspid regurgitation after isolated left sided valve surgery: a systematic review and meta analysis. Cardiology. 2014 Nov;129(4):242-9.
30. Matsuyama K, Matsumoto M, Sugita T, Nishizawa J, Tokuda Y, Matsuo T. Predictors of residual tricuspid regurgitation after mitral valve surgery. Ann Thorac Surg. 2003 Jun;75(6):1826-8.
31. Kim HK, Kim YJ, Kim KI, Jo SH, Kim KB, Ahn H, et al. Impact of the maze operation combined with left sided valve surgery on the change in tricuspid regurgitation over time. Circulation. 2005 Aug;112 Suppl9:S14-9.
32. Wang G, Sun Z, Xia J, Deng Y, Chen J, Su G, et al. Predictors of secondary tricuspid regurgitation after left sided valve replacement. Surg Today. 2008 Aug;38(9):778-83.
33. Porter A, Shapira Y, Wurzel M, Sulkes J, Vaturi M, Adler Y, et al. Tricuspid regurgitation late after mitral valve replacement: clinical and echocardiographic evaluation. J Heart Valve Dis. 1999 Jan;8(1):57-62.
34. Song H, Kang DH, Kim JH, Park KM, Song JM, Choi KJ, et al. Percutaneous mitral valvuloplasty versus surgical treatment in mitral stenosis with severe tricuspid regurgitation. Circulation. 2007 Sep;116 Suppl11:S246-50.
35. Bezdah L, Allouche E, Chabchoub S, Sidhom S, Ben Ahmed H, Ouchtati W, et al. Predictors of functional tricuspid regurgitation after successful left-sided valve surgery. Arch Cardiovasc Dis. 2018 Jan;10(1):80.

36. Nathalie P. Guide du parcours de soins: maladie rénale chronique de l'adulte (MRC) 2021 [On line]. HAS [cited 05/12/2023]; Available from URL: . https://wwwhas-sante.fr/upload/docs/application/pdf/2021-09/guide__mrc.pdf
37. Marwick TH, Amann K, Bangalore S, Cavalcante JL, Charytan DM, Craig JC, et al. Chronic kidney disease and valvular heart disease: conclusions from a kidney disease: improving global outcomes (KDIGO) controversies conference. Kidney Int. 2019 Oct;96(4):836-49.
38. Samad Z, Sivak JA, Phelan M, Schulte PJ, Patel U, Velazquez EJ. Prevalence and outcomes of left sided valvular heart disease associated with chronic kidney disease. J Am Heart Assoc. 2017 Oct;6(10):e006044.
39. Boudoulas H. Etiology of valvular heart disease. Expert Rev Cardiovasc Ther. 2003 Nov;1(4):523-32.
40. Come PC, Riley MF. Tricuspid anular dilatation and failure of tricuspid leaflet coaptation in tricuspid regurgitation. Am J Cardiol. 1985 Feb;55:599-601.
41. Sagie A, Schwammenthal E, Padial LR, Vazquez de Prada JA, Weyman AE, Levine RA. Determinants of functional tricuspid regurgitation in incomplete tricuspid valve closure: doppler color flow study of 109 patients. J Am Coll Cardiol. 1994 Aug;24(2):446-53.
42. Essayagh B, Antoine C, Benfari G, Maalouf J, Michelena HI, Crestanello JA, et al. Functional tricuspid regurgitation of degenerative mitral valve disease: a crucial determinant of survival. Eur Heart J. 2020 May;41(20):1918-29.
43. Navia JL, Brozzi NA, Klein AL, Ling LF, Kittayarak C, Nowicki ER, et al. Moderate tricuspid regurgitation with left sided degenerative heart valve disease: to repair or not to repair? Ann Thorac Surg. 2012 Jan;93(1):59-67.
44. Habib G, Lancellotti P, Antunes MJ, Bongiorni MG, Casalta JP, Del Zotti F, et al. 2015 (ESC) guidelines for the management of infective endocarditis: the task force for the management of infective endocarditis of the european society of cardiology (ESC). Endorsed by: european association for cardio thoracic surgery (EACTS), the european association of nuclear medicine (EANM). Eur Heart J. 2015 Nov;36(44):3075-128.
45. Aaron MD, Abadie J, Abuzeid WM, Adamolekun B, Adigun CG, Alexandrov AV, et al. MSD manual for professionals: New York heart association (NYHA) heart failure classification [online]. MSD [cited 05/12/2023]; Available à URL: https://www.msdmanuals.com/fr/professional/multimedia/table/classification-of-heart-failure-of-the-new-york-heart- association-nyha
46. Rodriguez Gabella T, Voisine P, Dagenais F, Mohammadi S, Perron J, Dumont E, et al. Long term outcomes following surgical aortic bioprosthesis implantation. J Am Coll Cardiol. 2018 Apr;71(13):1401-12.

47. García Fuster R, Vázquez A, Peláez AG, Martín E, Cánovas S, Gil O, et al. Factors for development of late significant tricuspid regurgitation after mitral valve replacement: the impact of subvalvular preservation. Eur J Cardiothorac Surg 2011 Jun;39(6):866-74.
48. Von Alvensleben JC. Syncope and palpitations. Pediatr Clin North Am. 2020 Oct;67(5):801-10.
49. Park SJ, Enriquez Sarano M, Chang SA, Choi JO, Lee SC, Park SW, et al. Hemodynamic patterns for symptomatic presentations of severe aortic stenosis. JACC Cardiovasc Imaging. 2013 Feb;6(2):137-46.
50. Fan Y, Pui Wai Lee A. Valvular disease and heart failure with preserved ejection fraction. Heart Fail Clin. 2021 Jul;17(3):387- 95.
51. Maganti K, Rigolin VH, Sarano ME, Bonow RO. Valvular heart disease: diagnosis and management. Mayo Clin Proc. 2010 May;85(5):483-500.
52. Matsunaga A, Duran CM. Progression of tricuspid regurgitation after repaired functional ischemic mitral regurgitation. Circulation. 2005 Aug;112 Suppl9:S453-7.
53. Sanfilippo AJ, Abascal VM, Sheehan M, Oertel LB, Harrigan P, Hughes RA, et al. Atrial enlargement as a consequence of atrial fibrillation. A prospective echocardiographic study. Circulation. 1990 Sep;82(3):792-7.
54. Henry WL, Morganroth J, Pearlman AS, Clark CE, Redwood DR, Itscoitz SB, et al. Relation between echocardiographically determined left atrial size and atrial fibrillation. Circulation. 1976 Feb;53(2):273-9.
55. Je HG, Song H, Jung SH, Choo SJ, Song JM, Kang DH, et al. Impact of the maze operation on the progression of mild functional tricuspid regurgitation. J Thorac Cardiovasc Surg. 2008 Nov;136(5):1187-92.
56. Bouchahda N, Kallala MY, Zemni I, Ben Messaoud M, Boussaada M, Hasnaoui T, et al. Left atrium reservoir function is central in patients with rheumatic mitral stenosis. Int J Cardiovasc Imaging 2022 Dec;38(6):1257-66.
57. Benjamin EJ, D'agostino RB, Belanger AJ, Wolf PA, Levy D. Left atrial size and the risk of stroke and death. The framingham heart study. Circulation. 1995 Aug;92(4):835-41.
58. Kizer JR, Bella JN, Palmieri V, Liu JE, Best LG, Lee ET, et al. Left atrial diameter as an independent predictor of first clinical cardiovascular events in middle aged and elderly adults: the strong heart study (SHS). Am Heart J. 2006 Feb;151(2):412-8.
59. Vaturi M, Sagie A, Shapira Y, Feldman A, Fink N, Strasberg B, et al. Impact of atrial fibrillation on clinical status, atrial size and hemodynamics in patients after mitral valve replacement. J Heart Valve Dis. 2001 Nov;10(6):763-6.
60. Tager R, Skudicky D, Mueller U, Essop R, Hammond G, Sareli P. Long term follow up of rheumatic patients undergoing left sided valve replacement with

tricuspid annuloplasty validity of preoperative echocardiographic criteria in the decision to perform tricuspid annuloplasty. Am J Cardiol. 1998 Apr;81(8):1013-6.
61. Takano H, Hiramatsu M, Kida H, Uenoyama M, Horiguchi K, Yamauchi T, et al. Severe tricuspid regurgitation after mitral valve surgery: the risk factors and results of the aggressive application of prophylactic tricuspid valve repair. Surg Today. 2017 Apr;47(4):445-56.
62. Colombo T, Russo C, Ciliberto GR, Lanfranconi M, Bruschi G, Agati S, et al. Tricuspid regurgitation secondary to mitral valve disease: tricuspid annulus function as guide to tricuspid valve repair. Cardiovasc Surg. 2001 Aug;9(4):369-77.
63. Demirbag R. Management of the tricuspid valve regurgitation. Anadolu Kardiyol Derg. 2009 Jul;9 Suppl1:S43-9.
64. Taamallah K, Jabloun TY, Guebsi M, Hajlaoui N, Lahidheb D, Fehri W. Subclinical right ventricular dysfunction in patients with mitral stenosis. J Echocardiogr. 2022 Jun;20(2):87-96.
65. Van De Veire NR, Braun J, Delgado V, Versteegh MIM, Dion RA, Klautz RJM, et al. Tricuspid annuloplasty prevents right ventricular dilatation and progression of tricuspid regurgitation in patients with tricuspid annular dilatation undergoing mitral valve repair. J Thorac Cardiovasc Surg. 2011 Jun;141(6):1431-9.
66. Desai RR, Vargas Abello LM, Klein AL, Marwick TH, Krasuski RA, Ye Y, et al. Tricuspid regurgitation and right ventricular function after mitral valve surgery with or without concomitant tricuspid valve procedure. J Thorac Cardiovasc Surg. 2013 Nov;146(5):1126-32.
67. Vargas Abello LM, Klein AL, Marwick TH, Nowicki ER, Rajeswaran J, Puwanant S, et al. Understanding right ventricular dysfunction and functional tricuspid regurgitation accompanying mitral valve disease. J Thorac Cardiovasc Surg. 2013 May;145(5):1234-41.
68. Haq IU, Haq I, Griffin B, Xu B. Imaging to evaluate suspected infective endocarditis. Cleve Clin J Med. 2021 Mar;88(3):163-72.
69. Denault AY, Couture P, Beaulieu Y, Haddad F, Deschamps A, Nozza A, et al. Right ventricular depression after cardiopulmonary bypass for valvular surgery. J Cardiothorac Vasc Anesth. 2015 Aug;29(4):836-44.
70. Cormier B, Lansac E, Obadia JP, Tribouilloy C. Valvular heart disease in adults. Paris: Lavoisier; 2014.
71. Muthialu N, Varma SK, Ramanathan S, Padmanabhan C, Rao KM, Srinivasan M. Effect of chordal preservation on left ventricular function. Asian Cardiovasc Thorac Ann. 2005 Sep;13(3):233-7.
72. Unger P, Pibarot P, Tribouilloy C, Lancellotti P, Maisano F, Iung B, et al.

Multiple and mixed valvular heart diseases. Circ Cardiovasc Imaging. 2018 Aug;11(8):e007862.
73. Yang LT, Enriquez Sarano M, Scott CG, Padang R, Maalouf JF, Pellikka PA, et al. Concomitant mitral regurgitation in patients with chronic aortic regurgitation. J Am Coll Cardiol. 2020 Jul;76(3):233-46.
74. Kalra R, Patel N, Doshi R, Arora G, Arora P. Evaluation of the incidence of new onset atrial fibrillation after aortic valve replacement. JAMA Intern Med. 2019 Aug;179(8):1122-30.
75. Jatene MB, Marcial MB, Tarasoutchi F, Cardoso RA, Pomerantzeff P, Jatene AD. Influence of the maze procedure on the treatment of rheumatic atrial fibrillation evaluation of rhythm control and clinical outcome in a comparative study. Eur J Cardiothorac Surg. 2000 Feb;17(2):117-24.
76. Lagier D, Fischer F, Fornier W, Huynh TM, Cholley B, Guinard B, et al. Effect of open lung vs conventional perioperative ventilation strategies on postoperative pulmonary complications after on pump cardiac surgery: the (PROVECS) randomized clinical trial. Intensive Care Med. 2019 Oct;45(10):1401-12.
77. Kollef MH, Sharpless L, Vlasnik J, Pasque C, Murphy D, Fraser VJ. The impact of nosocomial infections on patient outcomes following cardiac surgery. Chest. 1997 Sep;112(3):666-75.
78. Xiao P, Song W, Han Z. Characteristics of pulmonary infection after mitral valve repair in patients with metabolic syndrome and its relationship with blood pressure, blood glucose and blood lipid. Exp Ther Med. 2018 Dec;16(6):5003-8.
79. Riera M, Ibáñez J, Herrero J, Ignacio Sáez De Ibarra J, Enríquez F, Campillo C, et al. Respiratory tract infections after cardiac surgery: impact on hospital morbidity and mortality. J Cardiovasc Surg. 2010 Dec;51(6):907-14.
80. Hall TS, Brevetti GR, Skoultchi AJ, Sines JC, Gregory P, Spotnitz AJ. Re exploration for hemorrhage following open heart surgery differentiation on the causes of bleeding and the impact on patient outcomes. Ann Thorac Cardiovasc Surg. 2001 Dec;7(6):352-7.
81. Fang ZA, Navaei AH, Hensch L, Hui SKR, Teruya J. Hemostatic management of extracorporeal circuits including cardiopulmonary bypass and extracorporeal membrane oxygenation. Semin Thromb Hemost. 2020 Feb;46(1):62-72.
82. Kuvin JT, Harati NA, Pandian NG, Bojar RM, Khabbaz KR. Postoperative cardiac tamponade in the modern surgical era. Ann Thorac Surg. 2002 Oct;74(4):1148-53.
83. Uzun K, Günaydin ZY, Tataroglu C, Bekta§ O. The preventive role of the posterior pericardial window in the development of late cardiac tamponade

following heart valve surgery. Interact Cardiovasc Thorac Surg. 2016 May;22(5):641-6.
84. Canádyová J, Zmeko D, Mokrácek A. Re exploration for
bleeding or tamponade after cardiac operation. Interact Cardiovasc Thorac Surg. 2012 Jun;14(6):704-7.
85. Kristensen KL, Rauer LJ, Mortensen PE, Kjeldsen BJ. Reoperation for bleeding in cardiac surgery. Interact Cardiovasc Thorac Surg. 2012 Jun;14(6):709-13.
86. Merin O, Ilan M, Oren A, Fink D, Deeb M, Bitran D, et al. Permanent pacemaker implantation following cardiac surgery: indications and long term follow up. Pacing Clin Electrophysiol. 2009 Jan;32(1):7-12.
87. Ferrari ADL, Süssenbach CP, Guaragna JCVDC, Piccoli JDCE, Gazzoni GF, Ferreira DK, et al. Atrioventricular block in the postoperative period of heart valve surgery: incidence, risk factors and hospital evolution. Rev Bras Cir Cardiovasc. 2011 Jul;26(3):364-72.
88. Viles Gonzalez JF, Enriquez AD, Castillo JG, Coffey JO, Pastori L, Reddy VY, et al. Incidence, predictors, and evolution of conduction disorders and atrial arrhythmias after contemporary mitral valve repair. Cardiol J. 2014 May;21(5):569-75.
89. Nascimento CS, Viotti Júnior LA, Silva LHF, Araújo AM, Bragalha AMLA, Gubolino LA. Bloqueio atrioventricular de alto grau induzido pela cirurgia cardíaca: estudo de critérios de reversibilidade. Braz J Cardiovasc Surg. 1997 Jan;12:56-61.
90. Gummert JF, Barten MJ, Hans C, Kluge M, Doll N, Walther T, et al. Mediastinitis and cardiac surgery an updated risk factor analysis in 10,373 consecutive adult patients. Thorac Cardiovasc Surg. 2002 Apr;50(2):87-91.
91. Braxton JH, Marrin CAS, McGrath PD, Morton JR, Norotsky M, Charlesworth DC, et al. 10 year follow up of patients with and without mediastinitis. Semin Thorac Cardiovasc Surg. 2004 Jan;16(1):70-6.
92. Losanoff JE, Richman BW, Jones JW. Disruption and infection of median sternotomy: a comprehensive review. Eur J Cardiothorac Surg. 2002 May;21(5):831-9.
93. Di Mauro M, Bivona A, Iacò AL, Contini M, Gagliardi M, Varone E, et al. Mitral valve surgery for functional mitral regurgitation: prognostic role of tricuspid regurgitation. Eur J Cardiothorac Surg. 2009 Apr;35(4):635-9.
94. Chan V, Burwash IG, Lam BK, Auyeung T, Tran A, Mesana TG, et al. Clinical and echocardiographic impact of functional tricuspid regurgitation repair at the time of mitral valve replacement. Ann Thorac Surg. 2009 Oct;88(4):1209-15.
95. Li ZX, Guo ZP, Liu XC, Kong XR, Jing WB, Chen TN, et al. Surgical

treatment of tricuspid regurgitation after mitral valve surgery: a retrospective study in China. J Cardiothorac Surg. 2012 Apr;7:30.
96. Izumi C, Iga K, Konishi T. Progression of isolated tricuspid regurgitation late after mitral valve surgery for rheumatic mitral valve disease. J Heart Valve Dis. 2002 May;11(3):353-6.
97. W^sowicz M, Meineri M, Djaiani G, Mitsakakis N, Hegazi N, Xu W, et al. Early complications and immediate postoperative outcomes of paravalvular leaks after valve replacement surgery. J Cardiothorac Vasc Anesth. 2011 Aug;25(4):610-4.
98. Ruiz CE, Jelnin V, Kronzon I, Dudiy Y, Del Valle Fernandez R, Einhorn BN, et al. Clinical outcomes in patients undergoing percutaneous closure of periprosthetic paravalvular leaks. J Am Coll Cardiol. 2011 Nov;58(21):2210-7.
99. Dangas GD, Weitz JI, Giustino G, Makkar R, Mehran R. Prosthetic heart valve thrombosis. J Am Coll Cardiol. 2016 Dec;68(24):2670-89.
100. Gammie JS, Chu MWA, Falk V, Overbey JR, Moskowitz AJ, Gillinov M, et al. Concomitant tricuspid repair in patients with degenerative mitral regurgitation. N Engl J Med. 2022 Jan;386(4):327-39.
101. Zairi I, Mzoughi K, Saib W, Hannachi S. Predictive factors for the evolution of tricuspid insufficiency following left heart valve surgery. Cardiologie. tunis. [Online]. January 2016 [Accessed 5 December 2023]; 12(1):[7 pages]. Available at à the URL:
https://www.stcccv.org.tn/uploads/files/1505953776.pdf
102. Charfeddine S, Hammami R, Triki F, Abid L, Hentati M, Frikha I, et al. Tricuspid plasty: Carpentier annuloplasty versus De VEGA technique. Pan Afr Med J. June 2017;27:119.
103. Jeganathan R, Armstrong S, Alalao B, David T. The risk and outcomes of reoperative tricuspid valve surgery. Ann Thorac Surg. 2013 Jan;95(1):119-24.
104. Pfannmüller B, Moz M, Misfeld M, Borger MA, Funkat AK, Garbade J, et al. Isolated tricuspid valve surgery in patients with previous cardiac surgery. J Thorac Cardiovasc Surg. 2013 Oct;146(4):841- 7.

APPENDICES

Appendix 1: Data collection form

File number :
Full name :
Telephone number :
Service of origin :
Gender: 0. H 1. F
Age: Weight: Height: BMI :

Treatment in progress :

Aspégic: 0. no 1. yes Sintrom: 0. no 1. yes

Cardiovascular risk factors :

Tobacco: 0. No 1. Yes Hypertension: 0. No 1. Yes Dyslipidemia: 0. No 1. Yes Diabetes: 0. No 1. yes

Medical history :

Rheumatic fever: 0. no 1. yes
Percutaneous mitral dilatation: 0. no 1. yes
Créat: Chronic renal failure: 0. No 1. Yes Haemodialysis: 0. No 1. Yes
COPD: 0. No 1. Yes Stroke: 0. No 1. Yes
Coronary artery disease: 0. No 1. Yes Osteoarthritis: 0. No 1. Yes

Surgical history :

Cardiac surgery: 0. No 1. Yes; if yes Bypass surgery: 0. No 1. Yes RVAo: 0. No 1. Yes
RVM: 0. no 1. yes CMCF: 0. no 1. yes
Other surgical history: 0. no 1. yes
Euroscore II :
Emergency situation: 0. no 1. yes

Etiologies of valvulopathy :

Rheumatic: 0. No 1. Yes Degenerative: 0. No 1. Yes Endocarditis: 0. No 1. Yes
Bicuspidism: 0. no 1. yes Barlow's disease: 0. no 1. yes

Clinical examination :

Dyspnoea: 0. no 1. yes if yes NYHA :
Syncope: 0. No 1. Yes Lipothymia: 0. No 1. Yes
Angina: 0. no 1. yes
Palpitations: 0. no 1. yes
Fever: 0. No 1. Yes Auscultatory murmur: 0. No 1. Yes
Heart failure: 0. no 1. yes

Paraclinical examinations :

ECG :

AF: 0. No 1. Yes Conduction Tr: 0. No 1. Yes Repolarisation Tr: 0. No 1. Yes

Chest X-ray :

Cardiomegaly: 0. No 1. Yes Coil overload: 0. No 1. Yes Mitral silhouette: 0. No 1. yes

Preoperative TTE :

FeVG: DTDVG: Dilatation: 0. No 1. Yes Hypertrophy: 0. No 1. Yes
OG size: Dilatation: 0. No 1. Yes
OD size: Expansion: 0. no 1. yes

Aortic valve: 0. No 1. Yes Aortic surface: Aortic stenosis: 0. No 1. Yes Mean gradient: Aortic insufficiency: 0. no 1. yes
Mitral valve: 0. No 1. Yes Mitral stenosis: 0. No 1. Yes Mitral surface : Mitral insufficiency: 0. No 1. Yes Prolapse: 0. No 1. Yes
VD expansion: 0. No 1. Yes VD function: 0. No 1. Yes TAPSE: S': FR : PAPS: PAH: 0. no 1. yes
Grade of tricuspid insufficiency: AT size :

Preoperative TEE :

Left atrial thrombus: 0. No 1. Yes Vegetation: 0. No 1. No Abscess: 0. No 1. yes

Coronary angiography: 0. no 1. yes

ETSA: 0. no 1. yes

Operative gesture :

Clamping time :
CEC time :
Catecholamines: No catecholamines: 0. No 1. Yes Low dose: 0. No 1. Yes High dose: 0. no 1. yes
Mitral valve replacement: 0. no 1. yes Type of prosthesis :
Aortic valve replacement: 0. no 1. yes Type of prosthesis :
Combined gesture: 0. no 1. yes

Stay in intensive care :

Length of stay in intensive care :
Duration of intubation :
Antibiotics: 0. no 1. yes
Transfusion: 0. no 1. yes
Anticoagulation: Curative: 0. No 1. Yes Preventive: 0. No 1. Yes

Postoperative complications :

Postoperative bleeding: 0. No 1. Yes Resumption: 0. No 1. Yes
ACFA: 0. No 1. Yes BAV: 0. No 1. Yes Pace: 0. No 1. Yes Hypertensive peak: 0. No 1. yes
Tamponade: 0. no 1. yes Heart failure: 0. no 1. yes
Infectious lung disease: 0. No 1. Yes OAP: 0. No 1. Yes Reintubation: 0. No 1. Yes
Acute renal failure: 0. no 1. yes
Agitation: 0. no 1. yes
Parietal infection: 0. no 1. yes
Length of stay in intensive care :
Length of stay :
Immediate postoperative mortality: 0. no 1. yes

Remote monitoring :

Clinical :

Dyspnoea: 0. No 1. Yes NYHA stage :
Heart failure: 0. No 1. Yes Syncope: 0. No 1. Yes Lipothymia: 0. No 1. Yes
Chest pain: 0. no 1. yes

Ultrasound :

FeVG: DTDVG: Dilatation: 0. No 1. Yes Hypertrophy: 0. No 1. Yes

OG size: Dilatation: 0. No 1. Yes
OD size: Expansion: 0. no 1. yes
Aortic prosthesis: 0. No 1. Yes Stenosis: 0. No 1. Yes Leak: 0. No 1. Yes
Thrombosis: 0. no 1. yes
Mitral prosthesis: 0. No 1. Yes Stenosis: 0. No 1. Yes Leak: 0. No 1. Yes
Thrombosis: 0. no 1. yes
VD expansion: 0. No 1. Yes VD function: 0. No 1. Yes TAPSE: S': FR :
PAPS: PAH: 0. no 1. yes
Grade of tricuspid insufficiency: AT size :
Remote mortality: 0. No 1. Yes If yes, cause: Time :
Setback period :
Re-intervention: 0. no 1. yes if yes
Type of surgery :
Date of surgery :
Postoperative course :
Clinical monitoring: Ultrasound monitoring :

Appendix 2: NYHA stages of dyspnoea {Citation}

Classes and Stages of Heart Failure

The table below describes the different classes in the NYHA Functional Classification.

Class	Patient Symptoms
I	No limitation of physical activity. Ordinary physical activity does not cause undue fatigue, palpitation or shortness of breath.
II	Slight limitation of physical activity. Comfortable at rest. Ordinary physical activity results in fatigue, palpitation, shortness of breath or chest pain.
III	Marked limitation of physical activity. Comfortable at rest. Less than ordinary activity causes fatigue, palpitation, shortness of breath or chest pain.
IV	Symptoms of heart failure at rest. Any physical activity causes further discomfort.

Classes and Stages of Heart Failure

The table below describes the different classes in the NYHA Functional Classification.

Class Patient Symptoms

I No limitation of physical activity. Ordinary physical activity does not cause undue fatigue, palpitation or shortness of breath.

II Slight limitation of physical activity. Comfortable at rest. Ordinary physical activity results in fatigue, palpitation, shortness of breath or chest pain.

Ill Marked limitation of physical activity. Comfortable at rest. Less than ordinary activity causes fatigue, palpitation, shortness of breath or chest pain.

IV Symptoms of heart failure at rest. Any physical activity causes further discomfort.

Appendix 3: ASA classification

ASA Physical Status Classification System

1 Normal patient

2 Patient with moderate systemic abnormality

3 Patient with severe systemic abnormality

4 Patient with severe systemic abnormality representing a constant threat to life

5 Moribund patient unlikely to survive without intervention

6 These definitions are available in the annual edition of the ASA Relative Value Guide. There is no additional information to help classify patients.

Appendix 4: EACTS recommendations for surgery for of functional tricuspid insufficiency

Recommendations	Class[a]	Level[b]
Recommendations on tricuspid stenosis		
Recommendations on secondary tricuspid regurgitation		
Surgery is recommended in patients with severe secondary tricuspid regurgitation undergoing left-sided valve surgery.[423–427]	I	B
Surgery should be considered in patients with mild or moderate secondary tricuspid regurgitation with a dilated annulus (≥40 mm or >21 mm/m^2 by 2D echocardiography) undergoing left-sided valve surgery.[423,425–427]	IIa	B
Surgery should be considered in patients with severe secondary tricuspid regurgitation (with or without previous left-sided surgery) who are symptomatic or have RV dilatation, in the absence of severe RV or LV dysfunction and severe pulmonary vascular disease/hypertension.[418,433 e]	IIa	B
Transcatheter treatment of symptomatic secondary severe tricuspid regurgitation may be considered in inoperable patients at a Heart Valve Centre with expertise in the treatment of tricuspid valve disease.[f]	IIb	C

©ESC/EACTS 2021

Recommendations on tricuspid stenosis

Recommendations on secondary tricuspid regurgitation

Surgery is recommended in patients with severe
secondary tricuspid regurgitation undergoing left-sided valve surgery."-'[(3) (427)]
Surgery should be considered in patients with mild or moderate secondary tricuspid regurgitation with a dilated annulus (>40 mm or >21
mm/m^2 by 2D echocardiography) undergoing
left-sided valve surgery [(423)-(425)-127]
Surgery should be considered in patients with severe secondary tricuspid regurgitation (with or without previous left-sided surgery) who are symptomatic or have RV dilatation, in the absence of severe RV or LV dysfunction and severe pulmonary vascular disease/hypertension-.
sion.[(418)-433 c] I
Transcatheter treatment of symptomatic secondary severe tricuspid regurgitation may be considered in inoperable patients at a Heart Valve
Centre with expertise in the treatment of tricuspid valve disease.*

Summary

EVOLUTIONARY PROFILE OF TRICUSPID LESIONS AFTER LEFT HEART SURGERY: LONG-TERM RESULTS AND FACTORS ASSOCIATED WITH AGGRAVATION

Introduction :

Functional tricuspid insufficiency (TFI), often associated with left-sided valve damage, may spontaneously regress following repair of this valve disease. However, in other cases, it may worsen, necessitating repeat surgery. The objectives of our work were to study the evolution of unrepaired minimal to moderate TIA after left heart surgery and to identify the factors associated with the worsening of TIA after left heart valve surgery.

Methods :

This was a single-centre, descriptive, retrospective study, from January 2018 to December 2022, in the Cardiovascular Surgery Department of Abderrahmen Mami Hospital, including patients operated on for left-sided valve disease associated with minimal to moderate IT deemed non-surgical preoperatively.

Results :

A total of 57 patients were included. The mean age was 50.2 ± 13.9 years, with a clear predominance of women (63%). The majority of patients had more than two cardiovascular risk factors (37%). Atrial fibrillation (AF) was found in 29 patients preoperatively. Rheumatic disease was the main cause of valvular disease (75%). Preoperative echocardiography showed dilated left atrium (LA) in 51 patients (89%). Mitral valve replacement was the most common procedure (74%). Postoperatively, AF was present in 31 patients (54%). The mean follow-up time was 42.1 months. Late postoperative mortality was 3%. Late postoperative ultrasound showed that 15 patients (27%) had worsened their TIA to moderate to severe. Of these, five required redux surgery to repair the tricuspid defect (9%), while the other 10 were put on medical treatment (18%). We selected long-term anticoagulant treatment ($p = 0.008$), the presence of more than two risk factors ($p = 0.013$), preoperative AF ($p = 0.004$) and preoperative OG size > 33 cm2 ($p = 0.049$) as factors associated with worsening of CHF postoperatively.

Conclusion:

The worsening of TIA after left-sided valve surgery is a formidable complication, with a high morbidity and mortality rate. However, the indications for repairing a minimal to moderate TIA associated with left heart surgery remain controversial.

Key words: Heart valve replacement, Tricuspid insufficiency,
Right heart failure, Left atrium, Associated factors,
Evolution, Atrial fibrillation

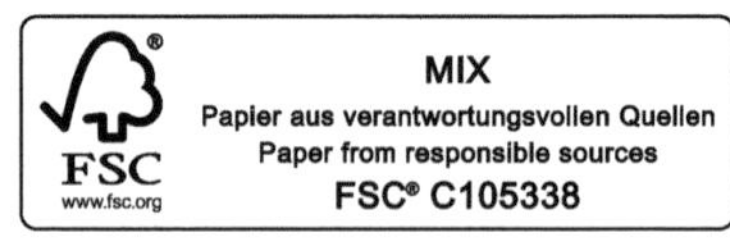

Printed by Books on Demand GmbH, Norderstedt / Germany